Understanding Assessment in Medical Education through Quality Assurance

Understanding Assessment in Medical Education through Quality Assurance

Bunmi Malau-Aduli, PhD
Associate Professor of Medical Education
Associate Dean of Learning and Teaching
College of Medicine and Dentistry
James Cook University, Douglas
Townsville, Queensland, Australia

Richard Hays
Professor of Remote and Rural Health
Medical Educator, Centre for Rural
and Remote Health
James Cook University
Mount Isa Hospital Campus
Joan/Deighton Street entrance
Mount Isa, Australia

Cees van der Vleuten, PhD
Professor of Education
Department of Educational Development
and Research
Faculty of Health, Medicine, and Life Sciences Maastricht University
Maastricht, The Netherlands

Mc
Graw
Hill

New York   Chicago   San Francisco   Athens   London   Madrid
Mexico City   New Delhi   Milan   Singapore   Sydney   Toronto

Understanding Assessment in Medical Education through Quality Assurance

1 2 3 4 5 6 7 8 9   LCR   26 25 24 23 22 21

ISBN 978-1-260-46965-3
MHID 1-260-46965-4

This book was set in Times NR MT Std by MPS Limited.
The editors were Kay Conerly and Teresa Massara.
The production supervisor was Catherine Saggese.
Project management was provided by Adwiti Pradhan.
The cover was designed by W2 Design.

Library of Congress Control Number: 2021942153

Contents

Chapter 1
Quality Assurance of Assessment Processes 1

Chapter 2
Roles and Responsibilities of Quality Assurance
Assessors 15

Chapter 7
The Role of Technology in the Quality Assurance of Assessment Processes 171

Chapter 8
Assuring Equivalence of Assessments across Settings . . 190

Chapter 9
Quality Assurance of an Assessment Program 217

Foreword

Trust is the most important aspect of health-care professionals' relationship with individual patients, their carers, citizens, and society. If trust is lost, then the system of care breaks down.

Patients need to be confident that their doctor, nurse, physiotherapist, or other health-care worker is competent to deliver the health care they need. Families and carers need to be reassured that their loved ones are safe, and societies need to be confident that the people who staff their health-care delivery systems are committed to providing safe, up-to-date, and appropriate treatment.

In 1998, in an article in the *BMJ*, Sir Cyril Chantler said

"Medicine used to be simple, ineffective, and relatively safe. It is now complex, effective, and potentially dangerous."

This statement is even more true today than in the last century. Ensuring that every graduate, medical trainee, and senior clinician is and remains competent to deliver increasingly technical and sophisticated health care is the responsibility of all medical educators.

However, the role of regulators in guiding educators and trainers and holding them to account for the competence of their graduates and practicing clinicians is gaining increasing prominence.

Consequently, assessing and assuring the competence of current and future medical graduates is of interest to everyone from patients to educators, regulators, employers and policy makers. This publication on the role of quality assurance in ensuring safe and competent health care for all is both necessary and timely, particularly in a period of unprecedented challenge such as the COVID-19 pandemic.

I recommend this publication for those who are involved in reviewing or providing existing educational programs to ensure the competence of their graduates and trainees and as an essential road map for those setting up new programs.

Trudie E Roberts
Professor of Medical Education,
University of Leeds, UK

Preface

Recent trends in medical education show an increased propensity towards competency-based education with increased reliance on assessment of mastery, entrustable professional activities, and milestones. Nonetheless, medical education is not exempt from the increasing societal expectations of accountability. Societal expectations make it imperative that medical educators adopt robust quality-assured assessment processes that are both fair and defensible.

This book aims to address a key gap in the literature by offering an international confluence of best practice in relation to quality assurance of assessment systems both within academic institutions and at the level of national and international accreditation. Although much is known about how to construct assessment practices that address assessment utility, there is less agreement on what should be explored when program, institutional, and jurisdictional assessment practices are examined by external regulators. Having a quality assurance guide that can be used across different medical programs and in different institutions across the globe would improve medical education assessment processes and practices as well as aid program development universally.

It is imperative to document evidence-based robust quality-assured assessment processes in order to guide medical institutions in developing internal monitoring processes that are vital to the ongoing improvement of the medical education they provide. In addition, accreditation agencies such as the General Medical Council, Australian Medical Council, Medical Council of Canada, and the American Medical Association have recently strengthened their standards and requirements around assessment because they recognize that assessment determines the quality of graduates. Quality assurance of assessment in medical education guarantees social accountability and quality improvement.

The planned approach is to provide international best practice through case studies. The chapters developed in this book are not intended to be prescriptive; they are solely to guide medical educators in improving the quality of their assessment processes and practices. The authors aim to inform, stimulate appraisal, and offer practical value by providing readers with case studies and examples of quality-assured assessment best practices.

B.S. Malau-Aduli

R.B. Hays

C.P.M. van der Vleuten

How to Use This book

Summary of Content	Contributors
Chapter 1 provides a general overview of the importance, principles, and mechanisms of assuring the quality of assessment processes in medical education.	Bunmi Malau-Aduli & Richard Hays
Chapter 2 discusses the functions of quality assurance (QA) assessors in facilitating evidence-based improvement of assessment practices.	Richard Hays & Bunmi Malau-Aduli
Chapter 3 presents the various aspects involved in the QA of written assessments.	Lambert Schuwirth, John Norcini, Leesa Walker, & David Prideaux
Chapter 4 utilizes the Kane Validity Framework to discuss QA mechanisms required for Objective Structured Clinical Examinations (OSCEs).	Katharine Boursicot, Sandra Kemp, & Richard Fuller
Chapter 5 focuses on the use and QA of Workplace Based Assessment (WBA) as part of a program of assessment within a medical education curriculum.	Karen Hauer, Jennifer Kogan, Patricia O'Sullivan, & Subha Ramani
Chapter 6 outlines the principles and rationale of programmatic assessment and discusses implications of the QA processes involved.	Lubberta H. de Jong, Harold Bok, Beth Bierer, & Cees van der Vleuten
Chapter 7 outlines the role of technology in the QA of assessment processes	Filipe Falcão, Patrício Costa, & José Miguel Pêgo
Chapter 8 discusses possible ways of assuring equivalence of assessment across diverse settings.	Tim Wilkinson &Vishna Devi Nadarajah
Chapter 9 discusses how quality of an assessment program can be assured in practice.	Lonneke Schellekens, Bert Slof, & Harold Bok
Chapter 10 discusses how assessment in medical education has changed in response to the recent disruption caused by the COVID-19 pandemic.	Richard Hays, Bunmi Malau-Aduli, Tim Wilkinson, & Cees van der Vleuten

▌TARGET AUDIENCE

This book is primarily of interest to medical educators, other health professions educators, postgraduate program educators, internal and external assessment evaluators, and administrators. Secondary audience is anyone else with an interest in assessment.

Editors

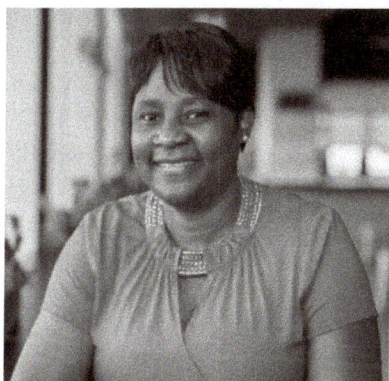

Bunmi S. Malau-Aduli, PhD, is the Associate Dean, Learning and Teaching and Academic Lead for Assessment and Evaluation at the College of Medicine and Dentistry, James Cook University, Queensland, Australia. She is also Co-Lead on the National Australian Collaboration for Clinical Assessment in Medicine (ACCLAiM). Her current medical education research interests include evaluation of learning and teaching, faculty development, examiner decision-making processes and quality assurance of assessment processes. She teaches into the undergraduate and postgraduate medical programs and leads the strategic development of program impact evaluation within the college. She facilitates and leads local, national, and international Item Writing and Assessment Workshops. She has more than 120 research publications in peer-reviewed scientific journals and supervises research students from diverse cultural backgrounds.

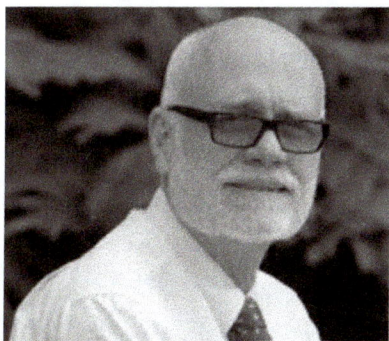

Richard B. Hays, PhD, MD, began his career in rural medicine, where his passion for medical education began with questions about how best to train and measure the performance of medical practitioners in underserved areas. He often works at the interface between education and clinical practice and has been involved in the development of several new or revised medical programs. He believes strongly that the most important part of curriculum development is optimizing assessment settings for and of learning. He has been a part of external QA processes in Australia, New Zealand, the United Kingdom, Ireland, Switzerland, China, Hong Kong, and North America.

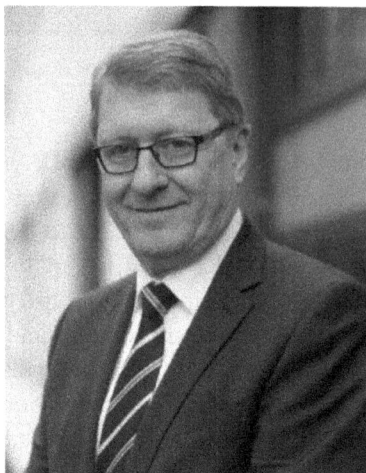

Cees P.M. van der Vleuten, PhD, has been at the University of Maastricht in The Netherlands since 1982. In 1996 he was appointed Professor of Education and Chair of the Department of Educational Development and Research in the Faculty of Health, Medicine, and Life Sciences (until 2014). Since 2005, he has been the Scientific Director of the School of Health Professions Education (until 2020). He mentors many researchers in medical education and has supervised more than 90 doctoral graduate students. His primary expertise lies in evaluation and assessment. He has published widely in this domain and holds numerous academic awards, including several career awards. In 2005, he received the John P. Hubbard Award for significant contribution to research and development of assessment of medical competence from the National Board of Medical Examiners in the United States. In 2010, he received a Dutch royal decoration for the societal impact of his work and in 2012 the Karolinska Prize for Research in Medical Education. He serves frequently as a consultant internationally. He holds honorary academic appointments in the School of Medicine, Flinders University, Adelaide, Australia; Western Sydney University, Sydney, Australia; the University of the Witwatersrand, Johannesburg, South Africa; the Uniformed Services University of the Health Sciences, Bethesda, Maryland, United States of America; and the University of California–San Francisco, San Francisco, United States.

Contributors

Bert Slof, PhD
Assistant Professor, Department of Education and Educational Sciences
Faculty of Social and Behavioral Sciences
Utrecht University

Beth S. Bierer, PhD
Associate Professor and Director of Assessment and Evaluation
Cleveland Clinic Lerner College of Medicine
Case Western Reserve University, United States
9500 Euclid Avenue—EC40, Cleveland, Ohio 44195, United States

Bunmi S. Malau-Aduli, BSc (Hons), MSc, PhD, Grad Cert ULT
Associate Professor of Medical Education, Associate Dean, Learning and Teaching
College of Medicine and Dentistry, James Cook University
Douglas, Townsville, Queensland 4811, Australia
Email: bunmi.malauaduli@jcu.edu.au

Cees P.M. van der Vleuten, PhD
Professor of Education, Department of Educational Development and Research
Former Scientific Director of the School of Health Professions Education
Faculty of Health, Medicine and Life Sciences, Maastricht University
P.O. Box 616 6200 MD Maastricht, The Netherlands
Email: c.vandervleuten@maastrichtuniversity.nl

David Prideaux, PhD
Emeritus Professor of Medical Education
Flinders Health and Medical Research Institute
Prideaux Health Professions Education
College of Medicine and Public Health, Flinders University
GPO Box 2100, Adelaide 5001, Australia

Filipe Falcão
Life and Health Sciences Research Institute (ICVS)
School of Medicine, University of Minho, Braga, Portugal
ICVS/3B's, PT Government Associate Laboratory, Braga/Guimarães, Portugal

Harold G.J. Bok, PhD
Associate Professor, the Department of Population Health Sciences
Faculty of Veterinary Medicine, Utrecht University, The Netherlands
Yalelaan 7 3584 CL Utrecht, The Netherlands

Jennifer R. Kogan, MD
Associate Dean for Student Success and Professional Development
Professor of Medicine, Perelman School of Medicine at the University of Pennsylvania
Perelman Center for Advanced Medicine
Building 421, Philadelphia, Pennsylvania 19104, United States

John Norcini, BA, PhD
Honorary Fellow of the Royal College of General Practitioners and
the Academy of Medical Educators, Research Professor,
SUNY Upstate Medical University, President Emeritus of FAIMER,
2607 W Darby Road, Havertown, Pennsylvania 19083, United States

José Miguel Pêgo, PhD
Associate Professor, Vice Dean
Life and Health Sciences Research Institute (ICVS)
School of Medicine, University of Minho, Braga, Portugal
ICVS/3B's, PT Government Associate Laboratory, Braga/Guimarães
Portugal. Postal code: 4710-057 Braga, Portugal

Karen E. Hauer, MD, PhD
Associate Dean for Competency Assessment and Professional Standards
Professor of Medicine, University of California, San Francisco
School of Medicine, 533 Parnassus Ave, U80
Box 0710, San Francisco, California 94143, United States

Katharine Boursicot, BSc, MBBS, MRCOG, MAHPE, NTF, SFHEA, FRSM
Associate Dean, Assessment & Progression
Duke–National University of Singapore Medical School
8 College Road, Singapore 169857

Lambert Schuwirth, MD, PhD, FANZHPE
Professor of Medical Education; Director, Flinders Health and Medical Research Institute
Prideaux Health Professions Education
College of Medicine and Public Health
Flinders University
GPO Box 2100
Adelaide 5001, Australia

Leesa Walker, MBBS, FRACGP, GDCE
Senior Lecturer, Flinders University
GPO Box 2100, Adelaide 5001, Australia

Lonneke L.H. Schellekens
PhD candidate, Educational Consultant and Trainer
PhD candidate, Department of Population Health Sciences Research
Faculty of Veterinary Medicine Utrecht University
Educational Consultant and Trainer, Centre of Educational Consultancy & Professional
Development Utrecht University, The Netherlands

Lubberta H. de Jong, MSc
PhD candidate at the Department of Population Health Sciences
Faculty of Veterinary Medicine, Utrecht University, The Netherlands
Address: Yalelaan 7 3584 CL Utrecht, The Netherlands

Patricia S. O'Sullivan, EdD
Director, Research and Development, Center for Faculty Educators
Professor of Medicine, University of California–San Francisco
School of Medicine, 533 Parnassus Ave, U80
Box 0710, San Francisco, CA 94143, United States

Patrício Costa
Life and Health Sciences Research Institute (ICVS)
School of Medicine, University of Minho, Braga, Portugal
ICVS/3B's, PT Government Associate Laboratory, Braga/Guimarães, Portugal

Richard B. Hays, MBBS, PhD
Professor of Remote and Rural Health, Medical Educator
Centre for Rural & Remote Health, James Cook University
PO Box 2572, Mount Isa Hospital Campus, Joan/Deighton Street entrance
Mount Isa QLD 4825, Australia
Email: richard.hays@jcu.edu.au

Richard Fuller, MA, MBChB, FRCP, FAcadMed
Consultant Geriatrician, Stroke Physician, and Vice-Dean of School of Medicine
at the University of Liverpool
Cedar House, Ashton St, Liverpool L69 3GE, United Kingdom

Sandra Kemp, BHMS(Ed), MA, PhD
Director of Learning and Teaching, Professor of Medical Education
Curtin Medical School, Curtin University, Building
410 Koorliny Way, Bentley, Perth, Western Australia 6102

Subha Ramani, MBBS, PhD, MPH
Associate Professor of Medicine, Harvard Medical School
Boston, Massachusetts, United States
Director of Evaluation and Scholars in Medical Education Pathway
Internal Medicine Residency Program, Brigham and Women's Hospital
75 Francis Street, Boston, Massachusetts 02115, United States

Tim J. Wilkinson, MBChB, MClinEd, PhD, MD, FRACP, FRCP, FANZAHPE, FAMEE
Professor of Medicine and Medical Education
Consultant Physician in Geriatric Medicine
Canterbury District Health Board, University of Otago, Otago, New Zealand

Vishna Devi Nadarajah, BSc (Hons), MHPE, PhD
Pro Vice-Chancellor Education & Institutional Development
International Medical University, Kuala Lumpur, Malaysia

Acknowledgments

Much love and gratitude to my husband (Enoch Malau-Aduli) and children (Fit Siji, Safat Page, and Senfat Paula Malau-Aduli) for their support over many years.

Bunmi S. Malau-Aduli

We would like to sincerely thank all our colleagues who have contributed to the book chapters. Your dedication, cooperation, and commitment to this work in the face of the COVID-19 pandemic were much appreciated. Such a major undertaking could have only been possible through effective team effort. Thanks also to the McGraw Hill publishing team, particularly Jim Shanahan, Teresa Massara, Kay Conerly, Catherine Saggese and Adwiti Pradhan for helping to materialize a major dream—the birth of this appealing book *Understanding Assessment in Medical Education through Quality Assurance*.

Bunmi S. Malau-Aduli
Richard B. Hays
Cees P.M. van der Vleuten

Quality Assurance of Assessment Processes 1

Bunmi S. Malau-Aduli and Richard B. Hays

CHAPTER HIGHLIGHTS

- This chapter provides a general overview of the importance and principles of quality assurance (QA) of assessment in medical education and emphasizes the need for continuous quality improvement of assessment practices and processes.
- QA is an inherent requirement and a process-oriented proactive approach to ensure the quality of assessment processes in medical education.
- Well-established internal and external QA processes are essential to foster institutional effectiveness, maintain continuous quality improvement, and promote accountability.
- QA of assessment processes empowers teaching staff to enhance the quality of the student learning experience and the "fitness for purpose" of graduates.

▍ ORIENTATION TO THE CHAPTER

Assessment is used by medical education provider institutions to improve learning outcomes and ensure accountability for learning and teaching practices. Although assessment goals and responsibilities involve administrators, educators, and students; improving learning for students lies squarely in the hands of educators, whose responsibility is to develop valid and reliable assessment instruments that both drive learning and provide evidence to stakeholders, such as employers, of the quality of education provided. Societal expectations make it imperative that medical educators adopt robust quality assured assessment processes that are both fair and defensible. This chapter begins with a general overview of the importance, rationale, and principles of QA of assessment in medical education. Next, it explores approaches and mechanisms of ensuring QA, using examples and case scenarios. Finally, the chapter concludes by emphasizing the significance and need for continuous quality improvement of assessment practices and processes.

▌INTRODUCTION

Assessment is a fundamental part of educational planning and curriculum delivery. Assessment serves the needs of three major groups—leaners, assessors, and regulators—each group may have different needs and perspectives but all of them should be included in QA processes. Therefore, it is pertinent that assessment instruction provided to students must be of high quality. The quality of learning and teaching is an essential component of educational quality and is associated with learning outcomes [1]. Subject experts need to develop and engage in appropriate assessment programs and practices that send the right signal to students about what and how they should be learning [2,3]. Ultimately, assessment tasks should be aligned with the course objectives and represent the course's intended learning outcomes [4,5], so that assessment reinforces learning the intended course outcomes

Understanding this curriculum alignment may be challenging. Are assessment practices determined by teaching practices or are teaching practices determined by assessment practices? If the two are aligned in the initial design, then they interact and shape each other symbiotically. Where changes are made to only one, the result can be chaotic, with limited success. **Case 1-1** is an example of an education provider who may well have had strong alignment between teaching and assessment practices, both rather "conservative" or "traditional." Teaching was not integrated across departments, and it assessed a series of independent courses, all of which must be "passed." The focus was on factual knowledge and judgment by senior faculty of clinical skills based on narrow samples. Professionalism, ethics, and articulating content ("putting everything together") were not assessed explicitly but were reflected in the judgments of the senior faculty. These are attributes of an institutional culture that is unlikely to change rapidly. Therefore, the example is one of trying to change too much too soon, even if the direction of change is sound. Assessment practices cannot easily become highly integrated, broadened, and implemented differently without changing the curriculum and perhaps the whole program. The education provider should have developed a plan for change that is agreed (ideally embraced enthusiastically) by faculty and students and implemented in stages, with milestones and review built in [6]. Educational expertise will be needed to inform the change, and resources may have to be reallocated to support the change. QA processes are likely to support both the changes and the change process, with realistic expectations about the scope of change and time frame. **Case 1-1** reflects a medical program in great difficulty if it does not pull back and prepare appropriately. There is some awareness of the challenges faced but uncertainty about how to proceed. Achieving change within institutions can be challenging, particularly without access to appropriate resources and amid a strong culture of following more traditional but not necessarily wrong teaching and assessment practices that are similar to those found in other higher education programs.

Case 1-1: Difficulty in Changing Institutional Culture

Education provider A was advised at the last accreditation cycle to consider changes to an assessment approach that featured a large number of 3-hour, 180-item, factual knowledge Multiple Choice Question (MCQs) run by strong departments and a small number of practical and clinical viva voce assessments in each major discipline and specialty. The program consists of several "courses" that are taught and assessed independently by each department, through which funding is distributed and research strengths mainly determine future funding and the promotion of academic faculty. Students must pass all assessments within each department to progress. Two academic staff members attended an international medical education conference and were impressed by the discussion on a more integrated approach and the concept of programmatic assessment. On their return, they obtained permission to implement substantial changes to assessment using a broader range of methods that integrated assessment across departments and specialties and changing the way that pass–fail decisions were made. However, the written submission indicated that the provider is struggling to achieve these changes. Departments are reluctant to cede control and, even though they agree in principle to the desire to update assessment practices, some plan to continue with their existing practices "until a better way is proven." The two "reformers" begin to realize the scale of the challenge that they face in achieving their goal.

RATIONALE FOR QUALITY ASSURANCE

Globally, concerns about QA in medical education have heightened in recent times. These concerns have heightened because of the need to produce excellent medical practitioners for safety and quality in health care delivery. Strategic partnership between the World Health Organization [7] and the World Federation for Medical Education (WFME) [8] sought to encourage the promotion of QA mechanisms and standards in medical education and served as a renewed stimulus for medical educational institutions to take a critical look at their QA mechanisms. Diverse interest groups and stakeholders are keenly interested in the quality of medical education. Therefore, a medical school or faculty must be accountable and consistent with the quality and caliber of training it provides. Medical schools need to have robust systems of ensuring quality in the implementation of curricula and the associated teaching and assessment activities that validate the learning process [9].

QA is an inherent requirement of assessment processes. However, QA and quality control (QC) have been used interchangeably. These terminologies are both important parts of managing quality but it is important to point out that they are not the same thing [10]. QC is a product-oriented reactive tool that focuses on identifying defects in the outcomes. Examples include requiring all vehicles with the same model name to look and function identically and all hamburgers from a particular franchise to look and taste identical. On the other hand, QA is a process-oriented proactive approach that focuses on ensuring quality in production systems. This is more appropriate to medical education, where the emphasis is on teaching, learning, and assessment processes that produce graduates who achieve equivalent outcomes at the point of graduation but then progress to many different potential career pathways that require continuing adaptation and development.

Murgatroyd and Morgan [11] (p. 45) defined QA as "the determination of standards, appropriate methods and quality requirements by an expert body, accompanied by a process of inspection or evaluation that examines the extent to which practice meets the standards." Similarly, Sallis [12] (2002) defined quality in medical education as acquiring prerequisite standards approved by external agencies and meeting these standards consistently. This exercise endeavors to intercept concerns before they occur and is related to processes rather than outcomes; that is, processes that portray and lead to social accountability and quality improvement. This implies medical educational institutions must develop and implement consistent institutional strategies to meet and enhance these standards mandated by external agencies. QA provides evidence to the public regarding institutional accountability and stewardship of resources. Using QA policies and procedures, institutions can self-evaluate or be subjected to external scrutiny in a regular, systematic, and substantive manner and thus provide evidence of the achievement of intended outcomes [13].

▌PRINCIPLES OF QUALITY ASSURANCE

The guiding principles of QA in assessment are highlighted in the purpose of assessment. The purpose of assessment is threefold and includes assessment to support learning, accountability and certification-progress-transfer [14]. Assessment to support learning refers to a progressive interaction between learning and assessment. This involves using assessment data to determine gaps, progress, and competency of learners to help improve learning and modify learning strategies. The assessment may be for decision-making (summative) or feedback (formative) purposes and is used to determine the degree of mastery attained in a subject. Assessment for accountability is an essential function of assessment and is the responsibility of educational programs to stakeholders (public and the government) for funding received, while assessment for certification, progress, and transfer ensures the employability and mobility of graduates as certification is required for employment [15].

The policies that govern QA of assessment are based on principles and conceptualizations. Different conceptualizations or principles have been reported in the literature. In the early 1990s, Harvey and Green identified the principles of QA as distinctive, consistent, transformative, value for money, and being fit for a specific purpose [16]. In more recent years, Schlinder et al. [17] identified four broad principles of QA that are consistent with previous research and these include: Quality being purposeful, transformative, distinctive, and accountable.

Using Harvey and Green's framework, the principles of QA in assessment for medical education can be classified into distinctive standards that are fit for purpose, value for money, and transformation. Setting distinctive standards in assessment refers to the establishment of credible, defensible, and acceptable standards in medical education [18]. When the quality of the assessment is distinctive, excellence is achieved through the fulfilment of set standards [17]. In addition, assessment should be fit for purpose. That means it should be an integrated model of assessment that optimizes both learning and decision-making functions in competency-based educational contexts [19]. It is imperative that assessment achieves set objectives and provides feedback to students to help them improve their learning [20]. Subsequently, when assessment improves learning, a positive transformation occurs in students' learning experiences, thus resulting in lifelong learning. In addition, educational institutions must remain accountable to stakeholders for the optimal use of resources and services provided [17]. Providing evidence that learning is promoted through aggregated learner results is a viable way to demonstrate accountability [15]. Other ways of providing accountability include international and national comparative benchmarking exercises [21]. Furthermore, resource allocation for assessment in medical education is inherently linked to accountability in terms of value for money, that is, return on investment [15,16].

Another important framework to consider in the QA of assessments in medical education is the Kane Validity Framework [22]. This framework provides a contemporary approach to collecting validity evidence for the interpretation or use of test scores. The framework proposes that a series of arguments and principles are required to determine the association between observed test takers' attributes and the assumed proficiency [22]. Application of the Kane Validity Framework in the QA of assessments is detailed in **Chapters 3 and 4**.

▌ APPROACHES TO QUALITY ASSURANCE

QA can be conducted in two major ways, regardless of the strategy used by an institution, it is important that evaluation demonstrates institutional effectiveness, fosters institutional improvement, and promotes accountability [23]. There are different approaches to QA. According to Kis [24], "there are three main approaches to QA: Accreditation, assessment and audit." Accreditation and assessment both monitor teaching and learning quality, whereas an audit focuses on a higher education institution's internal procedures. Accreditation is widely used by the Organization for Economic Cooperation and Development (OECD), and involves the evaluation of an institution or program against a standard threshold or requirement [24]. On the other hand, assessment is the graded evaluation of the outputs of a higher education institution, whereas a quality audit assesses the progress of the institution against its own set goals and objectives. There are two different methods of quality review: Internal and external reviews. *External quality review* refers to evaluations undertaken by individuals or bodies external to the program or institution [25]. In contrast, *internal quality monitoring* includes a wide range of services such as student and staff surveys, internal peer review of teaching, internal audits of quality procedures, surveys of recent graduates, and employers' views of graduates [24].

▌ QUALITY ASSURANCE MECHANISMS

QA may be either internal or external to a particular institution. The two mechanisms are usually separated, although the lines between the views may be blurred and each should inform the other. In several jurisdictions, each requires the other to be done and reports shared with both accreditation authorities. Detailed discussion of these mechanisms and the roles of QA assessors are presented in **Chapter 2**. In all reviews, the principles for how to approach the task are similar, as are the measurement tools that may be used. This information is presented in Table 1-1.

Table 1-1 QUALITY ASSURANCE MECHANISMS		
QA Mechanisms	**Examples**	**Measurement Tools**
External QA	Accreditation by medical education authorities Accreditation by higher education authorities	Written submissions Self-evaluations Commencement and completion data Student surveys and meetings Faculty surveys and meetings Observation of teaching methods Observation of examination processes Multiple campus visits National assessment results Postgraduate training outcomes Views of employers
Internal QA	Subject review Course review School or faculty review	Student survey or focus groups Subject survey Teaching evaluations Peer review of teaching Internal QA examiners External examiners

External Quality Assurance

External QA refers to the systems that are designed and operated by an external agency, often mandated by law, to monitor the quality of education provided by higher education institutions [26]. These external agencies may be professional, governmental, or quasi-governmental. Globally, the external QA mechanism adopted by countries for medical education is accreditation as recommended by the WFME [8], and institutions that have applied it have made significant positive impacts on their institutions internationally. Accreditation is a process whereby a mandated authority examines and appraises an educational institution using a set of distinctly outlined procedures and outcomes criteria [9]. The process involves establishing minimum standards, valuing institutional independence and academic freedom, and promoting continuous quality improvement. The standards of the major accreditation authorities are similar, including the same major themes or topics but with some structural and local contextual differences. Standards are reviewed periodically, and it is possible that new emphases emerge and provoke both anxiety and additional work in schools commencing a new accreditation cycle.

Case 1-2 is an example of a school that has previously met accreditation standards but now finds there may be gaps because the standards have changed while the program continued as before. This is not cause for either panic or arguing against new standards but an opportunity to check through self-evaluation where work is yet to be done to meet the new standards. The most important issue here is that program staff are aware of the changes and the work needed to meet the new standards. It is up to institutions to develop plans for change because they may require appointment of new faculty with relevant expertise or changes to resourcing. Accreditation authorities are likely to accept a clear plan to refine assessment practices to meet new standards, but there will be milestones and requirements at regular intervals (e.g., an annual report) for evidence of progress. **Case 1-2** reflects a medical program that is aware of the need for specific education expertise to respond to recent changes in accreditation standards.

Case 1-2: Responding to Changes in Accreditation Standards

Education provider B has an external accreditation exercise coming up, but the teaching leaders realize they do not have sufficient evidence to demonstrate quality of their training program, particularly in assessment. They do not believe that there is a problem with the graduates, who mostly do well, but after reading the current standards on assessment they realize that they do not have explicit blueprinting and standard-setting processes, features that have been added to the standards since the last accreditation cycle and are not mentioned in the broader institutional educational standards. Internal discussions focus on how important it is to meet current standards in the near future, balancing reputation with the profession and employers with potential loss of credibility with the accreditation agency. There is uncertainty about how much needs to change, so the leadership agrees to engage a credible senior medical educator to examine the assessment data, seeking evidence of any impact of current blueprinting and standard-setting practices, and to advise on what changes would strengthen their approach. This report was included as an appendix to the accreditation self-report submission, along with a plan for how to engage educational expertise to oversee development of improved practices over the next 2–3 years.

The purpose of accreditation in medical education is to encourage the social accountability of institutions for quality and guarantee for the value of medical education. The underlying principle of accreditation is meant to inspire institutions to initiate institutional mechanisms by which they would at least maintain and at best, seek to continuously improve the standards prescribed by the agency.

While external QA is usually contained within a particular national or regional jurisdiction, such as the United Kingdom, North America, Australia and New Zealand, medical education is becoming increasingly "globalized." Pressure is increasing to find ways of recognizing medical education programs across national and regional boundaries. Some nations have traditionally produced more graduates than needed domestically, expecting many to work in other nations. Other nations have traditionally relied on medical immigration to provide a workforce, particularly in smaller and more remote communities, raising ethical concerns [27]. Many new medical schools have been established to meet changing workforce needs due to increasing populations, ageing populations with more complex chronic diseases, and to "capture" a clinical workload base for the expansion of medical education [28]. Motivations vary from altruism around equivalence of opportunity and health outcomes to development of an "export industry" for profit. The outcome may be an increase in the number of medical graduates seeking to migrate.

The issues around recognizing educational quality are, of course, not limited to medical programs. **Case 1-3** is an example of a non-medical context. The program is generally regarded as sound. Students particularly like the pathway into employment because the last 2 years provide a basic salary to recognize that they contribute to team function as part of the health care workforce. Further, a substantial proportion of students are employed within the health service after graduation. On the other hand, students who do not secure longer-term employment feel disadvantaged when applying for positions elsewhere. Further, employers voice uncertainty about the additional supervision and "bedding in" period required for graduate from other health services. The accreditation process must address the question "Is there a problem here?" **Chapter 8** goes further into the issue of equivalence of assessment across several sites.

International health professional migration is a complex topic that is not within the scope of this book, except for its impact on the external QA of programs. There are variations across health professions, so it is essential to consult relevant authorities. For medicine, accreditation agencies are now collaborating on a process of recognition (or accreditation) of national or regional accreditation authorities through the WFME as driven by a 2016 objective of the World Health Authority [8]. The intention is that all graduates of medical programs that are accredited by a recognized national or regional accreditation authority will have an easier pathway to achieving recognition as a medical practitioner in every other nation with a recognized accreditation agency. This development has raised the profile of external accreditation, increased the number of

---

Case 1-3: Assuring Educational Quality across Training Sites

Education provider C provides the only program for a particular health profession within the jurisdiction. It does this by constructing a course that brings all students to study for years 1 and 2 to a central campus location, sharing resources with students in other health professional programs. Students are then allocated for the final 2 years to different health service employers throughout the jurisdiction. During these 2 years, students assume gradually increasing responsibility as team members, with Workplace Based Assessment (WBA) provided by both local and visiting clinical teachers who conduct similar assessment at several sites. Employers are especially happy with the quality of graduates from their own services, as all are familiar with local technology, people, and care pathways. However, they are wary about employing graduates embedded in other health services, where students are trained with different technologies and slightly different clinical pathways. Employers have a strong sense of ownership of "their" programs and prefer to employ only "their" graduates. A challenge for education provider C is therefore to demonstrate that the differences between the workplaces in which students are embedded has little or no impact on the quality of graduates and that all health service training sites produce graduates with equivalent learning outcomes and the ability to adapt to any new workplace environment.

---

external accreditations in many more nations, and increased the amount of external accreditation work happening around the world.

Internal Quality Assurance

The European Association for Quality Assurance in Higher Education (ENQA) [29] argues that an institution that has a well-established external QA mechanism but lacks strong internal QA, would not have significant improvement in overall quality. Internal QA is described as any activity and provisions carried out by an institution with a view to ensure educational quality. Institutional activities should include course evaluation, peer evaluation, and assessment. These activities would continuously enhance processes and quality outcomes for students. However, institutional activities may differ because of contextual differences in organizational, educational, socioeconomic, and other extenuating factors. The interplay of these factors (as described in **Case 1-2**) expose institutions to a myriad of challenges, including lack of funding to maintain or upgrade facilities, insufficient infrastructure, inadequate staff resources for teaching, administration, and information technology that may affect the quality of institutional outcomes. Nonetheless, this should not be a deterrent to implementing internal QA mechanisms, as such a decision may lead to periodic efforts to meet external agency standards. This may consequently impede improvements in processes, and in turn, have no real impact in terms of quality outcomes for students. This justifies the institutionalization of internal QA practices in medical educational institutions as an indispensable exercise, a process which goes beyond accreditation to develop and implement institution-specific strategies to ensure quality outcomes.

Approaches to internal QA vary across institutions and nations and may be highly contextual. In most nations, higher education is regulated and has its own external QA processes. These are often "light touch" processes that require education providers to conduct more robust internal QA at regular intervals, usually every few years. Panels will be appointed, including academics from other parts of the institution, chaired by a senior teaching and learning academic. A student may be included to provide their perspective. Sometimes an academic from another institution will be appointed to the panel to provide an external view to the internal review. These reviews are broad and based on how the particular institution applies national or regional policies in higher education. The relationship with national and international medical standards is likely to be weak because of the interface of graduation with workforce needs and readiness. In particular, assessment in medical education is often different from other higher education programs because of the strong focus on clinical assessment. In some nations, a strong tradition of external examiners exists. In such cases, an experienced medical academic may participate in varying aspects of assessment in medical programs, contributing a more informed external perspective to the internal QA processes [30].

Case 1-2 also demonstrates how higher education standards and medical education standards can have quite different emphases, particularly for assessment. Awareness of these differences is important in internal QA because the broader institution needs to understand that the context, requirements, and resourcing may need to be different even if there is no particular view on the details of assessment. Further, determining the extent of difference may be important in shaping the submission to the medical education QA authority. Internal QA should inform external QA by focusing on reviewing existing systems and procedures so that best practices can be exemplified and not-so-good ones can be identified and improved on with the promulgation of lessons learned and improvements made. There is no such thing as perfection in medical education and other education contexts. Robust internal QA processes help to raise key issues for review, thus minimizing the enormous amount of time spent during external QA processes.

AVOIDING COMMON PITFALLS

It is important to have a dedicated team or committee with expertise and in-depth knowledge of the curriculum, that oversees and ensures effective coordination of assessment QA processes within the faculty. Such a committee should be enabled to plan and implement necessary changes with regular ongoing review and improvement of assessment practices. Implementation of effective QA processes can be challenging and would require a well-defined communication strategy to engage all stakeholders. Ensuring shared understanding of the QA processes is the only way to achieve best practice. The following practical approaches can be used to avoid common pitfalls that could possibly be encountered while establishing assessment QA processes:

- Contextualize the QA process: You can't just copy what is done in other settings without considering the environmental context and determining how the internal assessment processes are linked.
- Avoid single perspective: Involve a range of stakeholders, including students as well as teaching, professional, and technical staff. Involving only people who design and implement the QA process may cause bias and limited scope of operation. Allowing scrutiny from other stakeholders creates an opportunity for continuous improvement.
- Develop a clear understanding of the purpose of the QA process at the start to provide guidance and focus on relevant goals and objectives. Such purpose statements can be reviewed regularly and revised (if required) to ensure currency of knowledge and foster best practice.
- Effectively communicate with and engage stakeholders in robust discussions to facilitate shared understanding and foster continuous improvement of practice.

CONCLUSION

Institutional structures and processes for QA add value in relation to pedagogical goals and objectives only if the connection to continuous improvement is transparent and unequivocal. The emphasis in medical education is on improving education processes that produce equivalent rather than identical graduates. To have any significance, QA frameworks must rely on people who are directly involved in the day-to-day operations of the assessment program. Assessment practices and teaching practices are inextricably linked and embedded within the organizational culture of an education provider. Standards in assessment change periodically and may differ from broader educational standards that may be applied to higher education institutions. Internal and external quality assurances are both important and should inform each other. The purpose of both internal and external scrutiny is to empower and inspire staff to fulfil their roles and obligations in order to enhance the quality of student learning experience and the "fitness for purpose" of graduates.

▌REFERENCES

1. Hanushek EA, Rivkin SG. Teacher Quality. In: Hanushek E, Welch F, eds. *Handbook of the Economics of Education*. Vol. 2. Amsterdam, Netherlands: Elsevier; 2006: 1051–1078.
2. Hays R. Assessment in Medical Education: Roles for Clinical Teachers. *The Clinical Teacher*. 2008;5(1):23–27.
3. Preston R, Gratani M, Owens K, Roche P, Zimanyi M, Malau-Aduli B. Exploring the Impact of Assessment on Medical Students' Learning. *Assessment & Evaluation in Higher Education*. 2019:1–16.
4. Biggs J. Aligning Teaching and Assessing to Course Objectives. *Teaching and Learning in Higher Education: New Trends and Innovations*. 2003:13–17.
5. Boud D, Falchikov N. Aligning Assessment with Long-Term Learning. *Assessment & Evaluation in Higher Education*. 2006;31(4):399–413. doi:10.1080/02602930600679050
6. Malau-Aduli BS, Zimitat C, Malau-Aduli AEO. Quality Assured Assessment Processes: Evaluating Staff Response to Change. *Higher Education Management and Policy*. 2011;23(1):1–24.
7. World Health Organization. About Quality Assurance. 2019. https://www.who.int/medicines/areas/quality_safety/quality_assurance/about/en/
8. World Federation of Medical Education (WFME). Accreditation. 2018. https://wfme.org/accreditation/
9. Norcini J, Anderson B, Bollela V, et al. 2018 Consensus Framework for Good Assessment. *Medical Teacher*. 2018;40(11):1102–1109. https://www.tandfonline.com/doi/abs/10.1080/0142159X.2018.1500016
10. Manghani K. Quality Assurance: Importance of Systems and Standard Operating Procedures. *Perspect Clin Res*. 2011;2(1):34–37. https://pubmed.ncbi.nlm.nih.gov/21584180/
11. Morgan C, Murgatroyd S. *Total Quality Management in the Public Sector*. Buckingham, UK: Open University Press; 1994.
12. Sallis E. *Total Quality Management in Education*. London, UK: Kogan Page; 2002.
13. Steadman DG. Accreditation Is Not School Accountability. *NASC Report*. 2001;13(2):4–51.

14. Newton PE. Clarifying the Purposes of Educational Assessment. *Assessment in Education*. 2007;14(2):149–170.

15. Archer E. The Assessment Purpose Triangle: Balancing the Purposes of Educational Assessment. *Frontiers in Education*. 2017;2(41). doi:10.3389/feduc.2017.00041

16. Harvey L, Green D. Defining Quality. *Assessment & Evaluation in Higher Education*. 1993;18(1):9–34.

17. Schindler LA, Puls-Elvidge S, Welzant H, Crawford L. *Definitions of Quality in Higher Education: A Synthesis of the Literature*. 2015. https://files.eric.ed.gov/fulltext/EJ1132898.pdf

18. Norcini JJ. Setting Standards on Educational Tests. *Med Educ*. 2003;37(5):464–469.

19. van der Vleuten CP, Schuwirth LW, Driessen EW, et al. A Model for Programmatic Assessment Fit for Purpose. *Medical Teacher*. 2012;34:205–214.

20. Hinett K, Knight P. Quality and Assessment. *Quality Assurance in Education*. 1996;4(3):3–10. doi:10.1108/09684889610125832

21. Archer E, Brown GT. Beyond Rhetoric: Leveraging Learning from New Zealand's Assessment Tools for Teaching and Learning for South Africa. *Education as Change*. 2013;17(1):131–147.

22. Kane MT. 2013. Validating the interpretations and uses of test scores. *J Educ Meas*. 50(1):1–73.

23. Baker RL. Evaluating Quality and Effectiveness: Regional Accreditation Principles and Practices. *Journal of Academic Librarianship*. 2002;28(1–2):3–7.

24. Kis V. Quality Assurance in Tertiary Education: Current Practices in OECD Countries and a Literature Review on Potential Effects. *Tertiary Review*. 2005;14(9).

25. Harvey L, Askling B. Quality in Higher Education. In: *The Dialogue Between Higher Education Research and Practice*. New York, NY: Springer; 2003: 69–83.

26. Matei L, Iwinska J. Quality Assurance in Higher Education: A Practical Handbook. Budapest, Hungary: Central European University, Yehuda Elkana Centre for Higher Education. 2016.

27. Mpofu C, Sen Gupta T, Hays R. The Ethics of Medical Practitioner Migration from Low Resourced Countries to the Developed World: A Call for Action by Health Systems and Individual Doctors. *Journal of Bioethical Inquiry*. 2016;3:395–406. https://doi.org/10.1007/s11673-016-9726-0

28. Hays RB, Strasser RP, Sen Gupta TK. Twelve Tips for Establishing a New Medical School. *Medical Teacher*. 2019. https://doi.org/10.1080/0142159X.2019.1571570

29. European Association for Quality Assurance in Higher Education (ENQA). 2010.

30. Hays RB, Bashford CL. The Role of External Examiners. *Clinical Teacher*. 2009;6:160–163.

Roles and Responsibilities of Quality Assurance Assessors

2

Richard B. Hays and Bunmi S. Malau-Aduli

CHAPTER HIGHLIGHTS

- This chapter raises the importance of assessment expertise and self-awareness among quality assurance (QA) assessors and highlights approaches to assessing quality against accreditation standards.
- Assessing quality against accreditation standards can be challenging as *accepted* practice may not be *best practice*.
- The complex nature of QA processes emphasizes the importance of multiple perspectives among QA assessors
- Constructive and timely feedback that is couched positively and details strengths and weaknesses in relation to specific standards can foster "buy-in" and shared understanding between QA assessors and the education provider.
- Being a QA assessor can contribute substantially to personal professional development as an educator and education manager.

❚ ORIENTATION TO THE CHAPTER

This chapter provides a general overview of the function of the QA assessor in facilitating self-evaluation and evidence-based improvement of assessment practices by education providers. The context is primarily that of medical programs, because they are often the most stringently applied by regulation authorities, but many other health professions have similar processes. Similarly, although framed mostly in the context of external QA, internal QA processes often require similar approaches, and experience here may boost confidence for newer external QA assessors. The chapter raises the importance of assessment expertise and self-awareness among QA assessors and highlights approaches to assessing quality against accreditation standards. Issues to consider in QA decision-making and the importance and delivery of constructive feedback are also discussed. Getting this balance right can be challenging as *accepted* practice might not be *best practice*. Feedback about how to approach best practice may inspire faculty in the relevant education provider, whereas criticism for not exceeding accepted practice may not be well received. QA processes work best when all participants share a common understanding of both the process and the work that is likely to be required. The chapter concludes by emphasizing the valuable and most important feature of the role of QA assessors. Case examples throughout the chapter serve as examples to illustrate key points about the roles and responsibilities of QA assessors.

▋ INTRODUCTION

Because assessment plays such a large role in learning, it is often the focus of external review. Almost regardless of what the curriculum and learning schedules include, or who teaches what, when and where, learners will focus on the what, how, when, and where of assessment because progressing through educational programs depends on passing whatever assessment hurdles are present. This learner behavior therefore makes assessment extremely important in any QA process. An external review usually happens in one of two ways. First, the education provider may appoint external examiners to contribute their views to routine internal QA processes, a practice that is common in the United Kingdom [1]. In this case, the benchmark is based on the experience of the external examiners in their own or other education providers. Second, external accreditation processes periodically review whole medical programs based on accreditation documents that have standards for each major aspect of medical education. Assessment is a substantial component of these standards, normally as a separate standard, with several criteria that represent desirable features of assessment. Most of this chapter relates to external assessment teams working under the auspices of accreditation authorities, but the principles are similar for individual external assessors engaged by the host education provider. An assumption is also made that the review is for a medical program within the same jurisdiction as the context is more similar than when reviewing a program in a different context [2].

At first glance, the roles and responsibilities of QA assessors in medical education may seem relatively simple. These are people with expertise in the field that is often based on qualifications, experience, or participation at several levels in medical education programs. They have been appointed by the host institution or relevant QA agency to sift through submissions from medical education providers and, in many jurisdictions, visit the institution to observe program delivery, seek confirmation of judgments, and further explore issues that may not be so clear. They then provide a judgment about how well the program meets expected standards. However, medical education is a complex field, and QA is a complex process, requiring opinions from multiple perspectives about a series of standards for which there are unlikely to be single best *gold standards* against which one *measures* program attributes and makes those judgments. Assessment is no different because there are many different assessment methods and many different ways to combine these methods to inform decisions about how successful the learning has been. Two aphorisms come to mind. The first is that "for every assessment question, there may be more than one correct answer" (Anonymous). The second is: "For every complex problem there is an answer that is clear, simple, and wrong" [3]. QA assessors need to look closely at assessment practices to reduce the likelihood of making judgments that may not truly reflect the impact on both student learning and graduates' work readiness or fitness to practice. This deep look should include what happens behind the more obvious features of setting and marking examinations. The performance of QA assessors may vary according to their specific backgrounds and training in QA processes, the quality and quantity of *evidence* provided, and the stance taken by both the medical program being quality assured and the QA agency. These issues are discussed further in this chapter and in **Chapters 6, 8, and 9**.

ASSESSMENT EXPERTISE AND SELF-AWARENESS IN QA ASSESSORS

Although external QA assessor team membership usually represents multiple perspectives—program managers (including deans), teachers, learners, health-care providers, and sometimes people from outside health professional roles (laypeople or health-care consumer representatives)—rarely are *experts* in assessment included. Ultimately, all team members have a voice in making judgments, and final outcomes are determined by the accreditation body, not the accrediting team. Although each team member may take the lead on writing reports on how well a program measures up against one or two standards, all team members should contribute their experiences and opinion to group discussion and judgment that are pitched more at the ordinary academic perspective on all standards. An obvious question arises: What is this *ordinary academic perspective*?

Although all faculties in a medical education provider institution are likely to be experienced in most aspects of teaching and assessment, perhaps with roles in managing teaching and assessment, it is less likely that they will have detailed knowledge of the theoretical basis for each standard. This is particularly true for standards in assessment, where what happens at the learner interface—on its own a complex process—should be supported by expertise in assessment methodology, design and the evaluation of assessment practices, ideally with an in-house *education office*. Just as much of this expertise will not be found in all faculty members involved in assessment of learners, QA assessors are also unlikely to be experts in assessment. All are likely to have been the subjects of assessment processes, most will have been assessors, and some will have managed assessment practices, but only a few will have formal qualifications and experiences in educational measurement. This breadth of expertise is particularly relevant when a sole external examiner is appointed by an institution to enhance internal QA processes, because ideally the whole assessment process is reviewed [1].

Deeper and narrower expertise can be a dual-edged sword. Although greater expertise can lead to judgments that reflect the best available evidence, it may also lead to "hawkish" judgments that may be more idealistic and ideological than practical in all health professional programs. Imagine what might happen if a QA team included only experts in each standard. Although programs that meet expert-judged standards may be good programs, the bar may be raised so high that many programs are judged as not meeting standards. The best approach is to assess what is happening currently, rather than what might happen, against the standards determined by the accreditation organization. These standards should reflect best available evidence when developed, be updated regularly and be accepted by participating educational institutions. Getting this balance right can be challenging, as *accepted* practice might not be *best practice*. Feedback about how to approach best practice may inspire faculty in the relevant education provider, whereas criticism for not exceeding accepted practice may not be well received. It may be better for any member of the team who has substantial assessment expertise to not be the primary assessor of the assessment standard, but rather a resource for the team to advise on current issues, allowing those with more general expertise to lead the discussion that achieves a balanced judgment.

▌INTERPRETING STANDARDS

All available medical education standards in use around the world share much in common. The World Federation of Medical Education (WFME) [4], the General Medical Council [5], the Australian Medical Council [6], and the Liaison Committee on Medical Education [7] are the most widely known, but many other jurisdictions have their own versions. All are similar, with separate standards for major components of medical education (e.g., governance, curriculum, assessment, student support, and research). Each standard has subheadings for sections, components, or criteria to guide judgment. The precise nomenclature and what is included under each heading may vary, but the scope of each set of standards is similar.

How open to interpretation are these standards? In theory, QA assessors should follow the letter and the spirit of the standards—a criterion-referenced approach—to improve consistency across accreditation team judgments. This both sets the bar for acceptable practice and provides common ground for guiding quality improvement, regardless of how well a program is achieving standards. An interesting feature of the WFME standards is that this principle is adopted explicitly. Each standard is expressed at two levels—one that meets currently acceptable standards and one that describes a higher level to guide quality development.

In reality, local jurisdictional norms will influence assessors—a form of localized norm-referencing modification—because inevitably assessors will be comparing the program with their own and with the others that they may have explored. Although this may be acceptable within jurisdictions where standards are similar across programs, care must be taken when applying standards internationally. The WFME standards are written for the developed world—relatively resource rich and with larger, more stable workforces and capacities for resource-intensive research. These standards may not translate so well if applied in developing nations [2]. Good examples include research performance and library resources. Ideally, QA assessors use standards designed for the specific jurisdiction in which they are working. More jurisdictions are adapting and developing their own versions of standards, usually based on the WFME standards that provide local contextual detail to what may be similar headline standards.

What to Look for in Judging Against Assessment Standards

Although it is unlikely that many faculty members will have substantial expertise in assessment methodology, design, and evaluation, arguably the most important asset to look for in a medical program with respect to assessment is access to that kind of assessment expertise. Some emerging issues in assessment may benefit from expertise in psychometrics, others from just discussing with peers elsewhere how best to manage similar issues. A list of topics that requires exploration, when considering how well assessment practices meet standards is provided in Table 2-1. This list is rather idealistic, although it may be a reasonable guide to the kind of evidence to be sought and the feedback that might be provided. Other sources of guidance include the websites of the relevant accreditation authority and the AMEE Aspire criteria [8,9]. It is important to check exactly what the relevant standards actually say and to follow those standards closely. Several of these topics are discussed in more detail in **Chapters 3, 4, and 5**.

A key principle underpinning assessment standards may be that the program faculty should be able to identify strengths and weaknesses,

TABLE 2-1   WHAT TO LOOK FOR IN JUDGING AGAINST ASSESSMENT STANDARDS
Is there constructive alignment—clear learning, assessment, or program outcomes? [10]
What is the governance of assessment—separate results management, anonymous decisions?
What are learners told about assessment and how are they informed?
How are assessment methods chosen, and do they cover the learning outcomes?
How are items developed, updated, reused, reviewed, and managed?
What is the level of learning being assessed (Miller's pyramid) [11]?
Is the approach programmatic, formative, or summative? [12]
What is the balance between assessment methods? [13]
How are individual tests set? Ask to see recent papers (securely).
What standard setting procedures are used? [14]
How are examiners trained? How many are trained?
How and to whom is assessment reported?
How are judgments made across individual test scores by results committees?
How are gaps in learning identified and remediated? [15]
How are changes in assessment decided and made?
How are appeals managed? [16]
How much *underground* assessment information is available?

have access to theory and evidence-based advice about options, and have the discussions needed to decide how assessment will be managed in this particular program. There may be more than one correct answer to every assessment question, depending on the specific context of the program. Variations in assessment practices compared to other programs are acceptable and offer opportunities to formally compare evaluations of assessment systems in more than one context [17], particularly if presented at education conferences or published in education journals. If QA assessors can be satisfied that the right questions about assessment practices have been considered and that relevant assessment expertise has facilitated appropriate discussions and decisions, they are more likely to consider assessment practices to be *acceptable practice*. **Case 2-1** presents a situation that is less than ideal and may result in adverse comments.

Case 2-1: Unacceptable Assessment Practice

After reading the submission presented by education provider A, questions were raised within the QA team about some details of the assessment practices. These questions were posed to the education provider as a request for more detailed information. The response was slow, arriving just before the site visit, and did not really answer the questions. During the site visit, the QA assessor team asked to meet with the assessment committee for clarification. During that meeting no one present could answer the questions. The chair said the committee did not have anyone on staff who could answer these questions but that they used proprietary external assessment software and had a part-time consultancy arrangement with an assessment "expert" who worked elsewhere. This individual was currently on 3 months' long service leave and was temporarily out of contact. The QA assessor team was left feeling quite unsure about the capacity of the education provider to develop and sustain appropriate assessment practices.

THE IMPORTANCE OF ASSESSMENT EXPERTISE WITHIN THE EDUCATION PROVIDER

All institutions providing medical programs should have on their staff list someone (ideally more than one) who has credible experience in these listed topics. Expertise in all is unlikely to be found in one person and more likely to be found in a range of management, academic, and technical staff members. Some of these may be in other parts of the university or available through collaborations with other medical programs. The balance of in-house expertise and external networks and consultations should be sufficient to ensure that assessment practices are consistent with learning and teaching practices. **Case 2-1** is an example of a potentially sound arrangement that appears to be fragile: Care should be taken to ensure that their appointed external expertise contributes and is available throughout accreditation processes. When purchasing proprietary external assessment software, care must be taken in balancing resources. It may be that the cost of the external software comes from reducing local education office staff numbers and expertise. Although external software can be helpful in both managing and quality assuring assessment practices (see **Chapter 9**), the responsibility for implementation and initial problem-solving is likely to be local. Ideally, a level of understanding of more complex issues, such as psychometrics, should be present within or readily accessible to the education provider; helpful resources are easily accessible [18,19].

ENHANCING THE SELF-EVALUATION OF THE EDUCATION PROVIDER

Education providers are required to provide a substantial amount of information for a desk audit by both the accreditation team secretariat and the QA accreditation team. Part of this submission is usually some form of self-evaluation of the program against the standards. This is perhaps the most interesting part of the submission, as it will make clear just how aware the faculty are of their strengths and weaknesses against the standards. Where weaknesses are not acknowledged (most programs have some), assessors have to explore carefully these mismatches in perception. Deliberate cover-up is less likely than poor self-awareness. **Case 2-2** is an example of poor self-awareness; this is uncommon but does happen occasionally. An important role of QA assessors then is to support the development of self-awareness, ideally with consensus amongst faculty. This may be more likely to facilitate change within the education provider because self-awareness should increase motivation and ownership of any change process.

WHEN FURTHER EVIDENCE IS NECESSARY

Although further information will become available during the site visit, the better time to seek additional information may be after reading the submission and before the site visit. During the visit, there may not be sufficient time to absorb additional information, unless it is a response to

> **Case 2-2: Poor Self-Awareness**
>
> Education provider B has a well-established medical program that had been delivered for about 200 years. The submission for the current accreditation cycle appears to be "cut and paste" from previous submissions. The outcome of the last cycle was that there was an outdated, highly traditional curriculum, reliance on small numbers of highly subjective clinical assessments, and weakness in student support systems. These issues are mentioned only briefly in this submission, with little indication of improvement, even though employers had concerns about the quality of the graduates and the student society independently approached the accreditation agency about persisting concerns. The tone of the submission was "We have been doing this for much longer than the accreditation authority has existed, and we believe that we know better." The accreditation authority was contacted and made high-level contact with the education provider to seek more appropriate engagement.

a specific request, as QA assessors have to keep a great deal of information at the forefront of their thinking for the duration of the site visit. The quality of writing in the submission becomes important here because the best submissions are written specifically for the accreditation process, with sections that address every standard, explain the basis of the self-evaluation, and list relevant evidence as either hypertext links or appendices. The evidence cited could be intranet sites, subject guides, policy documents, minutes of meetings, published papers, and so on. Ideally, the key information from each source is summarized in the submission, with clear directions to where specific additional information can be found. This allows assessors to obtain an overview of the evidence base and dip in and out of the more detailed documents.

Should a possible source of information not be listed or appended, assessors should seek that information, ideally well before the site visit, through the accreditation organization from the education provider. Please note that these requests can be met with frustration because the information may well be in the submission somewhere, although perhaps linked poorly to the particular standard or section. It is not uncommon for education providers to place huge amounts of information as appendices but not necessarily help with navigation, leaving it to readers to work out for themselves what to read and where to find it. This approach results in much more work for the QA assessors and can increase frustration levels in both QA assessors and education providers.

Most accreditation cycles require providers to include details of planned significant changes that will take place during the next accreditations cycle. These include curriculum revision, cohort increases, and commissioning of additional clinical training facilities. These may well be desirable changes that are well supported by funders, employers, and local authorities. They may pose no threat to program standards—and may even improve them. However, the details should be provided in advance to the accreditation body rather than "sprung" on accreditation teams, as the current program will be delivered and "run out" for a few years yet. The major issues will be additional resourcing, potential distraction of faculty, and perception of *abandonment* by students in the current program. **Case 2-3** is an example of how the provider addresses both the current program and future initiatives in advance. Even if the approval of the future initiatives is not the task of the accreditation team, clarity is provided around the separation of current program from major new initiatives.

Case 2-3: Addressing Current and Future Program Initiatives

Education provider C had a 45-year history of providing medical education that had previously met all education standards. At the time of the current accreditations cycle, plans were in place to increase student numbers by 30% to meet the needs of a population increase and expansion of the health-care system. These additional students would be at the main campus for the first half of the program and then based in a new clinical campus 100 km away. This required substantial investment by both the education provider and the health-care system management, appointment and training of more faculty, installation of a stronger information technology system including video-conference equipment for both teaching and management, a "refreshed" curriculum, and changes to assessment practices to increase reliance on Workplace Based Assessment (WBA) at dispersed sites. The education provider prepared a comprehensive submission that addressed all standards for the current program and separately addressed the planning for the expansion, including details of finances, plans for staffing, managing the curriculum and assessment development, timelines, and managing foreseeable risks. This allowed the QA team to address the important question; "Does this program meet current standards?" and to feel confident that the proposed expansion could be achieved without compromising the standards.

WHEN REQUIRED ACTION IS NECESSARY

In most cases, findings that suggest weakness or raise concerns about a standard will be met with an open and honest discussion with faculty members. Nobody gets everything perfectly correct all of the time and faculty are likely to be aware of where they could make improvements, ideally even suggesting to the QA assessors where improvements could be made. This is a sign of a *healthy* learning organization and contributes to an engaging QA process that results in agreement between the QA assessor team and the education provider. Occasionally, there is resistance and the process becomes more adversarial than collegial. In this situation, the QA assessor team leader should contact the accreditation organization for advice. There may be a history of conflict arising from past accreditation reports, resulting in raised sensitivity to criticism or even resistance to accept "outside interference." Tensions can usually be defused through discussions, but if a major concern needs to be addressed, managing it becomes an issue for more senior managers.

DECISION-MAKING IN QUALITY ASSURANCE

By the end of the accreditation process, QA assessor teams are required to make decisions about how well the relevant program meets accreditation standards. There are three major issues to consider in this decision-making. First, any decision must relate to the documented standards and be supported by evidence. Ideally, more than one source of information or evidence should be sought before any judgment is made. For example, if students report concerns about a particular assessment practice, it is important to look at what the students are told about their assessments (the intranet, discussion with other students and faculty) and to look at the assessment reporting data (results, pass rates, examiner training, etc.). The outcome may be that the concern is confirmed, but it may also be just a view of a loud minority based on a specific incident. **Case 2-4** is an example of such an incident. One reason why each QA assessor should contribute to discussions about all standards is that this makes it more likely that different perspectives and sources of information will be encountered. Team meetings allow for multiple sources of information to be brought into discussions and resulting judgments. Usually, the team reaches a consensus for each judgment. This triangulated validation provides a much stronger foundation on which to make judgments and will strengthen the feedback provided about quality improvement. QA assessors are unlikely to accept a single source of concern, unless it is potentially critical to meeting a standard. As with assessing a portfolio, credibility and dependability are the main considerations, using a mixture of quantitative and qualitative information [20].

Case 2-4: Making Decision on Reported Concerns

In the weeks prior to an accreditation team visit, the accreditation authority receives a submission from some students complaining of a higher than usual failure rate of students in year 1 because of errors within the assessment office. This issue also featured in local media, leading to a degree of public discussion. The students demanded a meeting with the accreditation team to air their concerns. With the permission of the provider, the issue was explored during meetings with students, faculty, and the assessment office. Blueprinting and standard-setting procedures were reviewed. The outcome was that all except a small number of failed students were content and indicated that assessment practices were appropriate, although appeal and remediation processes were not as clear as they should be. This judgment was communicated to the education provider and was used later to support a defense in the local media.

The second issue is the internal consistency of judgments within standards. Each standard has several different sections, components, or criteria, and individual judgments must be made about each section, component, or criterion. It is not uncommon for parts of a standard to be judged as suboptimal, but how does this affect the judgment about the overall standard? The outcome may vary, depending on the relative weight of the weaknesses. In some cases, the weakness may be judged to be significant (hence judged as not met) but that the overall standard is met and could be improved if the unmet component were addressed.

The third issue is that, QA assessor teams are not the final decision-makers,—that is, the role of the committee managing accreditation. The QA assessors provide confirmed, factual information about what is happening on the ground, what seems to either meet or not meet the standards, and recommendations about how to improve the program. The accreditation committee reviews the report and either accepts or amends the judgments and recommendations. Amendments are likely to reflect information that the QA assessor team does not have, such as correspondence about past accreditation reports or changes to accreditation policies or national education or workforce strategies. This distancing of the QA assessors from the final decision should encourage QA assessors to be honest and open about their findings, comfortable in the knowledge that final decisions will reflect rather than necessarily adopt their own judgments.

THE IMPORTANCE OF FEEDBACK AND HOW TO DELIVER FEEDBACK

It is essential that any criticism be constructive, with feedback that is couched positively and is related to specific standards, details what might be strengths or weaknesses, and is timely. These feedback attributes are similar to those recommended for all feedback processes [21] even though evidence for change after feedback is mixed. Although timeliness may seem not to be in the hands of the QA assessor team, because final reports may not come for several weeks after the accreditation committee has completed the task and the organization has approved the report for release, it is important that the education program leader (usually the dean) is made aware of the likely outcomes by the end of the site visit. In some jurisdictions, an oral summary is provided to staff at the host education provider at the end of the visit. This means that the team's judgments about strengths and weaknesses and likely areas where changes may be either recommended or required should be determined before the site visit concludes and be provided (usually verbally) to the program leader. There are two reasons for this. First, accreditation organizations usually prefer a *no surprises* approach whereby education providers know what is likely to be in the final report and have time to consider their response. Second, it's an opportunity for the accreditation team to gauge the likely response of the education provider. QA processes may work best when all participants share a common understanding of both the process and the work that is likely to be required. Although uncommon, there have been examples of education providers reacting strongly to accreditation reports, even threatening legal action if reputations are damaged. Some providers hold senior program managers accountable for accreditation reports that are not *excellent*, and some have lost their positions. If a strong reaction appears likely, the QA team leader should advise the accreditation organization.

WHO LEARNS THE MOST FROM PARTICIPATION IN QA PROCESSES?

General agreement holds that in many cases of observation of performance, the observer learns more than the observed [22,23]. Although this is not proven in the larger scale accreditation processes, the situation is likely to be similar. People being observed are under pressure, having overworked to prepare the submission and participate in the site visit while maintaining concurrent implementation of a complex medical program. Some may feel that their jobs are at risk if the report is less than what the education provider expects. On the other hand, QA assessors have an interesting opportunity to see how others grapple with issues that may be quite similar to those affecting their own program. They may see other ways of dealing with challenges and take back new or broader perspectives, to their own workplace. Being a QA assessor can contribute substantially to personal professional development as an educator and education manager [24]. This supports the view that QA assessment teams should include relative newcomers to QA processes as a longer-term strategy to build and share accreditation expertise.

▌AVOIDING COMMON PITFALLS

Being a QA assessor is hard work. The cognitive load of carrying so much information at the front of mind is considerable. Getting away from normal work duties for several days can be difficult, particularly for more senior program managers. It is easy to arrive poorly prepared and to be distracted by major events at the usual work place. It may be tempting to make firm judgments before all information is considered. It is easy to compare constantly with one's own program, resulting in two potential errors. First, is to think that anything other than what you are familiar with is wrong, resulting in resistance to different or new ways. Second, is to think that what you are seeing is much better than you are used to and thus to be focused on concerns about your own program or role. Personal expertise can result in bias towards the best rather than accepted practice. It may also be easy to become frustrated if responses to previous recommendations or requirements for change have not happened in timely manner. Achieving change within organizations can be difficult, even in our own institutions, let alone other organizations that we may not understand as well. Table 2-2 lists some suggestions for avoiding these potential pitfalls.

▌CONCLUSION

Being a QA assessor in the field of assessment combines opportunities and responsibilities with hard work. The perspectives of learners, assessment candidates, assessors, assessment managers, and users of health care are important and should be considered. There are opportunities for personal and professional growth as learning from what others do is valuable, whether successful or not. On the other hand, it is demanding work with a high cognitive load that is often additional to normal work requirements. An underpinning philosophy of continuing quality improvement is important, with (or with access to) appropriate assessment expertise,

TABLE 2-2   AVOIDING PITFALLS
Do the prereading and approach the task with a clear head and impressions rather than a firm view.
Minimize distractions caused by texts, calls, and emails from outside. Turn devices off and check them only during breaks.
Seek actively and listen to the perspectives of different groups within the provider and within the team.
Focus on what the standards say.
Avoid comparison with one's own program.
Avoid applying narrow personal expertise as the benchmark. There is rarely only a single correct answer.
Be open to different or new ways of doing things.
Recognize and praise things that are done well.
Be aware that changes can be difficult and slow. There may be a good explanation for why a concern has not improved since an interim report a year ago.
Try to identify barriers to change and facilitate finding solutions.
Utilize a *no surprises* approach in communicating with the education provider team.

but also openness to different or new ways. Sharing of practice is a valuable process, particularly for the QA assessors, but also to develop a shared understanding of accepted practice. Practice that is better than *accepted* should be recognized and praised. Sometimes, triangulated evidence points to a need for some difficult feedback and significant decisions about requirements for change. How to balance assessment expert advice; the perspectives of patients, learners, assessors, and managers; and an understanding of local constraints and opportunities may be the most important feature of the role.

▌ REFERENCES

1. Hays RB, Bashford CL. The Role of External Examiners. *The Clinical Teacher*. 2009;6:160–163.
2. Hays RB. The Potential Impact of the Revision of the Basic World Federation Medical Education Standards. *Medical Teacher*. 2014;36(6):459–462.

3. Mencken HL. Quotes. BrainyQuote.com; n.d. https://www.brainyquote.com/quotes/h_l_mencken_129796

4. WFME. *Basic Medical Education WFME Global Standards for Quality Improvement. The 2015 Revision.* France, Denmark: World Federation for Medical Education; 2015. https://wfme.org/download/wfme-global-standards-for-quality-improvement-bme/

5. General Medical Council. *Promoting Excellence: Standards for Medical Education and Training*; 2015. https://www.gmc-uk.org/education/standards.asp

6. Australian Medical Council Limited. Standards for Assessment and Accreditation of Primary Medical Programs by the Australian Medical Council. Kingston, ACT: Australian Medical Council Limited; 2012. https://www.amc.org.au/files/d0ffcecda9608cf49c66c93a79a4ad549638bea0_original.pdf

7. Liaison Committee on Medical Education. *Functions and Structure of a Medical School*; 2020. www/lcme/org/

8. Association of Medical Education in Europe. *Areas of Excellence: Assessment of Students*; 2021. https://www.aspire-to-excellence.org/Areas+of+Excellence/

9. Hunt D, Klamen D, Harden RM, Ali F. The ASPIRE-to-Excellence Program: A Global Effort to Improve the Quality of Medical Education. *Acad Med.* 2018;93(8):1117–1119. doi:10.1097/ACM.0000000000002099. PMID: 29261539

10. Biggs JB. *Teaching for Quality Learning at University.* 2nd ed. Buckingham, England: Open University Press/Society for Research into Higher Education; 2003.

11. Miller GE. The Assessment of Clinical Skills/Competence/Performance. *Academic Medicine.* 1990;65:S63–S67.

12. Van Der Vleuten CPM, Schuwirth LWT. Assessing Professional Competence: From Methods to Programmes. *Medical Education.* 2005;39:309–317. https://doi.org/10.1111/j.1365-2929.2005.02094.x

13. Norcini J, Anderson B, Bollelo V, et al. 2018 Consensus Framework for Good Assessment. *Medical Teacher.* 2018. https://doi.org/10.1080/0142159X.2018.1500016

14. Cizek GJ, Bunch MB. *Standard Setting: A Guide to Establishing and Evaluating Performance Standards on Tests.* Thousand Oaks, CA: Sage Publications; 2007.

15. Hays RB. Remediation and Reassessment in Undergraduate Medical School Examinations. *Medical Teacher.* 2012;34(2):91–92.

16. Hays RB, Hamlin G, Crane L. 12 Tips: Increasing the Defensibility of Assessment. *Medical Teacher.* 2015;37:433–436.

17. Malau-Aduli BS, Teague P-A, Turner R, et al. Improving Assessment Practice Through Cross-Institutional Collaboration: An Exercise on the Use of OSCEs. *Medical Teacher.* 2016;38(3):263–271. https://doi.org/10.3109/0142159X.2015.1016487

18. Bloch R, Norman GR. Generalisability Theory for the Perplexed: A Practical Introduction and Guide. *Medical Teacher* (AMEE Guide No. 68). 2015;960–992. https://doi.org/10.3109/0142159X.2012.703791

19. De Champlain AF. A Primer on Classical Test Theory and Item Response Theory for Assessments in Medical Education. *Medical Education.* 2010;44:09–117. https://doi.org/10.1111/j.1365-2923.2009.03425.x

20. Driessen E, Van Der Vleuten C, Schuwirth L, Van Tartwijk J, Vermunt J. The Use of Qualitative Research Criteria for Portfolio Assessment as an Alternative to Reliability Evaluation: A Case Study. *Medical Education*. 2005;39:214–220. https://doi.org/10.1111/j.1365-2929.2004.02059.x
21. Bing-You R, Hayes V, Varaklis K, et al. Feedback for Learners in Medical Education: What Is Known? A Scoping Review. *Academic Medicine*. 2017, September;92(9):1346–1354. https://doi.org/10.1097/ACM.0000000000001578
22. Tenenberg J. Learning Through Observing Peers in Practice. *Studies in Higher Education*. 2016;41:756–773. doi:10.1080/03075079.2014.950954
23. Saad SL, Richmond CE, Jones K, Malau-Aduli BS. Manifold Benefits from Quality Assurance in Clinical Assessment. *Medical Education*. 2021. https://doi.org/10.1111/medu.14484
24. Saad SL, Richmond CE, Jones K, Malau-Aduli BS. Developing a Community of Practice for Quality Assurance within Healthcare Assessment. *Medical Teacher*. 2020. doi:10.1080/0142159X.2020.1830959

3 Quality Assurance of Written Assessment

Lambert Schuwirth, John Norcini, Leesa Walker, and David Prideaux

CHAPTER HIGHLIGHTS

- Quality assurance in written tests not only is important for the validity and defensibility of the outcomes but also leads to improved organizational expertise.
- The quality of written items mainly depends on two aspects: the creativity, relevance, and engaging nature of the content, and the adherence to item construction rules to minimize false positive and false negative responses.
- Even when the outcome of the assessment may be numerical or quantitative scores, quality cannot be quantified. If quality relates to issues such as creativity, relevance, and the mitigation of item construction flaws it is by nature a so-called shared narrative.

▮ ORIENTATION TO THE CHAPTER

Regardless of whether a medical school uses a more traditional assessment program or a programmatic assessment approach, there is likely to be a component that uses written assessment. For the assessment program as a whole, to lead to defensible, credible and fair decisions, all its components need to be of good quality, because both passing and failing students unjustly is detrimental.

Deciding whether a student is ready to progress is not the only purpose of assessment. Essential for education is the provision of feedback and guidance on learning, so these are important aspects of assessment as well.

What all these purposes have in common is that they require a good assessment program, and this cannot be guaranteed without a rigorous process of quality assurance. This chapter presents the various aspects involved in quality assurance specifically tailored to written assessment.

INTRODUCTION—PURPOSE OF ASSESSMENT

Assessing students is not a goal in itself; it is always done for a specific purpose. The quality of an assessment activity therefore starts with a clear understanding of its purpose. Purposes can firstly be defined in terms of the consequences—what the assessment is trying to achieve.

The most obvious purpose is to determine whether the learner or candidate has achieved a satisfactory level of competence, skills, knowledge, and so on. This can be an important determinant in whether a candidate is ready to enter medical school, progress to the next phase in learning, or graduate and care for patients.

Assessment will also drive student study behavior and learning. The content of the assessment, the type of assessments, when they are administered, and the rules and regulations around them will have an impact on students' study behavior [1–3]. Although we sometimes chide students for being assessment driven, this reaction is natural and has always been the case. Consequently, we need to ensure that content, format, programming, and regulatory structure are such that they drive students' study behavior in the desired direction. For example, because continuous learning leads to better uptake, retention, and access to learned material than block learning, more continuous assessment programs are preferable with or without final examinations.

Assessment not only drives study behavior but also drives learning. With *learning* we mean the type of activities that students undertake to engage with the subject matter. An example of how assessment is being used to steer student learning is the concept of assessment *for* learning [4,5]. In assessment for learning programs, the way the student takes up the feedback and incorporates it in future learning and progress are intrinsic aspects of the assessment program. Thus, the purpose of assessment for learning is not only to drive study behavior to facilitate learning but also to help the student develop a feedback-seeking and applying attitude.

Finally, assessment can be used to provide the organization with information as to the quality of the study program. There are many ways in which assessment information can be combined and collated to provide such program evaluation information. For example, if items in an examination sample an important component of the curriculum but are answered incorrectly by a large group of students, then the curriculum or teaching may need revision.

The purpose of the assessment can also be framed in terms of what it tries to assess. In some cases, this is straightforward. If, for example, the assessment is aimed at judging whether students can take a patient's blood pressure, their performance can be directly observed and judged.

In most cases however, the assessment tries to assess something that is less directly observable. Competencies such as clinical reasoning, critical thinking, medical problem-solving, reflectivity, empathy, and so on are more elusive [6]. In those situations, it is important to be as explicit as possible about the nature of the purported competence. For example, an assessment that is designed to measure clinical reasoning requires a clear definition of *clinical reasoning* [7]. It can be seen as a process, a skill, an ability, an attitude or personality characteristic, and so on. With this we do not mean that a perfect definition of the competency is needed before it can be assessed but that sufficient agreement and shared subjectivity among the stakeholders concerning the competency is an important step in the quality assurance of assessment. Fundamentally, the challenge is that we are not able to directly observe what we want to assess, and so we must infer it from what we can observe, including student behaviors, writings, and other communications.

Once there is sufficient agreement on the purpose of the assessment, the next step is to determine how the assessment is going to capture that purpose and consequently, what the implications are for its design. In this part of the process, validity theory is helpful. A modern validity theory—Kane's validity theory—proposes that a series of rationales and arguments are needed to make the connection between observation (students' behaviors, writings, and other communication) and the assumed competency [8]. Kane's validity theory involves four steps of inferences: scoring, generalization, extrapolation, and implication. For this chapter, only the first two are relevant.

The first step is how to go from a set of observations to a score. Every assessment involves a series of observations—for example, how students tick boxes on MCQs or what they write in modified essay questions. Eventually, all these observations are summarized in a score, a grade, or a qualitative result. For validity reasons, this result must optimally represent the aggregate of all observations, and for this to be the case the following should be considered:

- Are all items relevant to the competency being assessed?
- Are all items quality controlled—that is, have all items been reviewed?
- Is the weighting of items proportional and necessary?
- Is there a blueprint and have the items been distributed according to the blueprint?
- Are the numbers of marks for each of the items proportional and defensible?
- Are the markers or raters sufficiently trained and briefed?
- Is the pass–fail score defensible, and have evidence-informed methods been used to set the standard?

The second inference is whether the score on the assessment sufficiently indicates the score students deserve based on their competence. Every assessment contains just a sample of a whole "universe" of possible items. Even a 200-item multiple-choice test is still only an $n = 200$ out of a "universe" of 10,000 to 100,000s of possible questions. For generalization, the following aspects should be considered:

- Is the number of items sufficient to be representative of the whole domain? In other words, is the reliability high enough?
- Is the number of examiners or markers sufficient to represent the whole domain of possible examiners and markers? If there are multiple markers available for open-ended questions, is the distribution of markers across the items efficient? For example, if a test consists of multiple essay questions and there are multiple markers available, from a reliability perspective it is more efficient to distribute the markers across items and not across students. This means that marker A marks essay 1 for all students, marker B marks essay 2 for all students, and so on. This way all students' total scores are based on multiple examiners.
- Is the number of occasions during which the assessment takes place sufficient to be representative? A single event is likely to be more influenced by unwanted variability than assessments over occasions; students can have good days and less good days, which will influence student performance on a single event. The good and not-so-good days, however, are more likely to average out over time.

▌FORMAT OF THE ASSESSMENT

In the design of assessment, the choice of the question format is often given more importance than it merits. This is often the starting point for lively debates and opinions or preferences around a particular format. In such discussions it is sometimes suggested that some question formats are unsuitable for certain competencies. The most popular example is the belief that multiple-choice items cannot test higher-order cognitive skills or clinical reasoning, reflection, critical thinking, or problem-solving. This, however, is largely a misconception. The literature on comparisons between different item formats generally agrees that the content of the question (what the question asks) is of overriding importance, whereas the format of the questions (how the response is captured) does not seem to play a meaningful role [9–13].

A more meaningful distinction is whether the item is patient or case based and asking for a decision on solutions specific to the presented case, or whether it is a factual knowledge orientation [14]. Case-based questions, whether open-ended or multiple-choice format, typically require the student to read the whole case; evaluate all the information; balance pieces of information against each other; generate, select, and prioritize hypotheses; and make a decision. Although an open-ended question may seem more suitable for this, there are many good examples in the literature of high-quality multiple-choice or other closed question types.

QUALITY ASPECTS IN THE ITEM WRITING PROCESS

Blueprinting

A blueprint is one aspect of quality assurance that is important to highlight [15]. A blueprint is a table or grid that stipulates how many of the questions will deal with each of the topics or domains on the test. It ensures content validity by guaranteeing that the distribution of items in the test is similar to the distribution of items in the curriculum or the clinical domain.

When creating a blueprint, avoid becoming too detailed. Sometimes, blueprints are created with several different dimensions; for example, disciplines (anatomy, physiology, pharmacology, etc.), domains (internal medicine, surgery, pediatrics, etc.), phases in life (neonatal period, early childhood, adolescence, adult, etc.), and many others. The more dimensions a blueprint has, the more complex the system becomes and the more challenging it is to fill each cell. For example, it may be especially difficult to write an item on surgical problems in the context of indigenous health in early childhood with pharmacological aspects or there may be fewer items on the test than cells in the blueprint. A blueprint is a plan for sampling from the domain, so there is virtue in keeping it as simple as needed for content representation.

Item Writing

Item writing as a creative design process

Most books on item writing start with a set of guidelines about what *not* to do when writing items. These guidelines are important, and we will deal with them later in the chapter. But before looking critically at flaws, there needs to be an *item*. Item writing is a creative design process, and it is often the most difficult part of test construction. Items need to be relevant, meaningful, and novel to some extent.

Having good and well organized knowledge is a necessary requirement for medical problem-solving [16,17]. However, this does not mean it is also a sufficient requirement for medical problem-solving. The medical education literature often discusses assessment of higher-order cognitive skills, application of knowledge, or clinical reasoning. Contrary to popular belief, MCQs are just as suited to the assessment of higher-order cognitive skills as open-ended questions. Questions that are asked in an appropriate context and present students with a problem while asking them for the solution trigger different thinking steps compared to rote factual knowledge questions. Examples of such questions are extended-matching items [18] or key feature approach items [19], although they can be cast as single-best-answer and open-ended questions as well.

In the production of such context-rich questions the following strategies may be helpful.

Whenever possible, use cases that are derived from real-life situations

Of course, the most intuitive source would be clinical cases, but basic science problems, public health problems, statistical problems, and methodological problems can all be used. It is essential, though, to have questions that are aimed at important decisions specific to the presented problems. Likewise, it is important to avoid uncommon presentations and uncommon problems.

The description of the information in the case must be as clear as possible

Start writing the case in question in the language with which you are most familiar. When you feel the case is complete, start rearranging the information in a logical order. In a patient case, this might be:

- What is your role?
- When and where are you seeing the patient?
- What is the patient's name, sex, and age?
- What are the results from history taking?
- What are the results from physical examination?
- Is there any additional pertinent information?

After this, remove any unnecessary jargon and any information that has already been medically preinterpreted (for example, *tachycardia* instead of a heart rate of 160 bpm).

Be sure to provide sufficient realistic discipline-specific information

It is important to ensure that all the information needed to answer the question is presented in the case. This not only means the information required to defend the correct answer but also information that makes other options defensibly incorrect. This will entail an iterative process in which your attention shifts from the writing of the question to the writing of the case.

Provide sufficient realistic contextual information

In a clinical case, for example, it is important to describe where you see the patient and whether you know more about the patient's history. The importance of contextual information pertains to more than just clinical cases. Public health, methodological, and statistical and basic science cases may also require relevant contextual information.

Provide sufficient negative information

It is also important to tell the student about findings that were not abnormal ("no rebound tenderness"). Avoid sweeping statements such as "otherwise normal." Everybody has their own routines, and with a sweeping statement the candidate will not know which procedures were performed and which were not.

Link the problems directly to the case

There is sometimes a temptation to write a case and then ask a question that is basically unrelated to it. This is inefficient; it takes time to write the case, and students need time to read the case even though it is irrelevant. Ensure that the questions asked cannot be answered without having read the whole case.

Focus on essential problems only

This is probably the most essential element of writing case-based items. Try to isolate the most essential decisions—the key features—of the case and focus your questions on those decisions. In clinical cases, this is often the diagnosis and treatment, but this is not always so. For example, in a rural primary care setting the decision whether to evacuate the patient may be more essential than the specific diagnosis.

Make sure all questions are phrased as clearly as possible to avoid any ambiguities

This is an issue that will be dealt with later in this chapter. However, it is important to realize that when there is a choice between more words and more clarity or fewer words and less clarity, the best choice is always more words and more clarity.

Other Creative Processes

Not always will it be possible to use real-life cases for the production of all items. In such cases, alternative strategies are available.

Transformation of information

As noted previously, it is rarely a good idea to randomly pick a piece of information from a textbook and ask a question about it. There is a risk that necessary contextual information will be lost or that what is being asked is simply not relevant or suitable for the assessment. On the other hand, there may be instances when it is helpful to use the literature as the basis for a question. Ebel [20] suggested the following strategies:

- Restate the concept in different words or paraphrase what was said in the literature.
- Restate parts of what was described in the literature.
- Ask for the opposite of what was described in the literature.
- Ask for the exceptions (if relevant).
- Ask for a relationship between the concept from the literature and other relevant concepts.
- Ask for possible implications or consequences of the concept.
- Ask for a problem situation in which the concept would need to be applied.

Six-Steps Approach

George Miller [21] suggested that writing items *de novo* is quite a complex task, so it is better to take the process step-by-step. He suggested the following steps:

- Select the information to be tested.
- Condense the information.
- Select the task on how the information is to be used.
- Write the item's stem.
- Write the answer.
- Write the distractors.

An alternative set of steps is:

- Define the area.
- Define the subject.
- Define the topic.
- Define the problem.
- Write the question in the easiest format.
- Write the question in the desired format.

Notebook Method

Although not everybody has access to actual practical problems (whether they are clinical or basic science problems), everybody may encounter situations that would be good starting points for a question. In those situations, it is advisable to record the event and the topics flowing from it. The traditional way of recording is a small notebook, but smartphones or tablets can be even easier. They can be stored as notes or as audio files. Typical triggering events would be:

- misconceptions of students,
- main points of lectures or other educational activities,
- points from your practice,
- your own random inspirations,
- results of your own additional study,
- patient or practice encounters, and
- discussion with family and friends (for example, as a trigger for items concerning professional behavior, ethics, or health economics).

Communities of Practice Approach

Although it is often difficult to organize meetings with people who have busy diaries, working together would be the fastest method of producing high-quality items. This meeting time is precious and should not be spent on trying to find suitable topics; that should be done before the meeting. It is better to use group time on the questions themselves, even if they are in rough form. Typically, other group members will be critical, challenging the accuracy and importance of the proposed items and offering refinements. These meetings do not have to be face-to-face but could easily be managed with online meeting platforms. In such meetings, the following list of activities is generally helpful:

- brainstorming about the questions,
- critiquing each other's questions,
- discussing the relevance of each question,
- checking the content using online or literature sources, and
- making notes of various solutions to item writing problems with a view of having a list of standard procedures for recurring item writing problems.

This chapter includes three case studies. The first case (**Case 3-1**) describes a change of assessment processes from one that relied almost entirely on end-of-year barrier exams to one that includes longitudinal assessment and the related requirements for quality assurance processes. The second (**Case 3-2**) describes a situation in which problems with the perceived relevance of items in a written assessment have to be solved. The third and final case (**Case 3-3**) reports on the lessons learned through the development of posttest quality assurance procedures.

Case 3-1: Making Changes to Assessment Processes	
Things to Consider	**Response**
What was the identified problem/need in your program relative to assessment?	A medical school decided to transition from one-off, end-of-year barrier examinations to longitudinal assessment, but this required more items to be written and the existing approach of organising 1-2 day item writing retreats was not sufficient for the required quantity and quality of item production.
What is the specifically needed assessment?	The new assessment program included progress testing and required four tests per year with items being released to students.
What did you create to address this need?	A small diverse group of clinicians and basic scientists was formed that met weekly to produce items for the test. Some items were sourced from old banks and divided among the group prior to meeting. Individuals would edit these items prior to the meeting. This included ensuring the item was up to date, had a relevant case and was clear. Where possible individuals would use this case to write other questions for inclusions in other tests. At each meeting individuals would present their items for group discussion and further refinement. Content expertise and further peer review was sourced from clinicians who were previously involved in the old assessments, in addition to flagging area that required more items.
What assessment principles were employed?	The principles of longitudinal assessment for better reliability, early detection of struggling students (with remediation) and optimising feedback to students by detailed results and release of items after the test.
What were the outcomes/lessons learned?	Change of assessment approach requires careful considerations and planning of the logistical requirements. High-quality assessment requires extensive quality assurance processes in place which are also able to produce the quantities needed. Such systems have to be in place before the change in assessment is implemented.

▌ THE DO'S AND DO NOT'S OF ITEM WRITING

When creative and relevant items have been produced, it is important that they enter a second round of quality assurance. Defining *quality* is not straightforward; it is a difficult concept to delineate. However, within your organization and your country it is important that there is a sufficiently shared view on what constitutes the quality of an item. This is especially important if a collaboration on item production or item exchange is taking place.

One quality indicator that can be more easily agreed on is whether an item is an optimal indicator for the presence or absence of the requisite competence or knowledge. In other words, each item should be a diagnostic test for "knowledge" or "competence." The implication of this is that high-quality items must be less likely to produce false-positive or false-negative results. With false-positive results, a candidate answers the item correctly or passes the test without having sufficient knowledge; false negative means the opposite. False-positive results typically occur when the item provides grammatical or logical cues, asks for commonsense knowledge, or allows the student to use certain test-taking strategies to find the answer without having the necessary knowledge. False negatives occur when the item is worded in a confusing way or suggests "deeper layers" that are not really there, in which case the more knowledgeable student is likely to overthink the item. There are ample examples of guidelines provided in various sources [22], and in this chapter we will summarize some of them.

There are numerous forms of written assessment methods, each with its own acronym, but they can be subdivided into categories based on either their stimulus or response format. Response formats are either a form of constructed-response types (open-ended types) or selected response types (closed question types). With respect to stimulus formats the question either asks for an isolated aspect or a decision in the context of a specific problem or case.

Constructed-response items

Constructed-response items comprise such formats as short-answer open questions, essays, and modified essay questions but can also mean report, theses, or modern information technology artefacts (narrated PowerPoints, videos, podcasts, etc.). There are several item construction suggestions that should be heeded when writing constructed-response items.

Ensure optimal clarity

The need for clarity pertains to every aspect of the question. First, students should be 100% clear on what is expected of them. For example, a question such as this is ambiguous with respect to wording:

– *What is the most important complication of a viral meningitis?*

Students are left with the dilemma of how to interpret the word *important*; does it relate to the most likely, the most frequent, the most severe, the most expensive to treat, or something else?

An item such as:

— *Name the most frequent complications of a viral meningitis?*

is unclear about how many answers are required and which complications belong to the category *most frequent*.

Second, there has to be clarity about the length of the answer. This is an issue with the following example:

— *Explain the etiology of viral meningitis*

There are whole textbook chapters on the etiology of meningitis, and it is probably not the intent of the question to require the student to write down a whole textbook chapter. But how long the answer should be is left in the dark. Another unwanted effect of this unclarity is that it invites students to apply a so-called blunderbuss technique; write down as much as they can in the hope that there will be sufficient correct information in the answer between incorrect bits of information. The solution is straightforward: Indicate the length of the answer, either in word count or number of lines, and be strict in the enforcement of that limitation.

Finally, it is necessary to be as clear as possible with respect to the level of detail or precision needed for the answer. For example, if a case is presented of a young boy with sudden onset of high fever, headaches, nuchal rigidity, and purpura and the question asks for the most likely diagnosis, the student may be unclear with respect to the levels of detail: *meningitis, bacterial meningitis, meningococcal meningitis.*

Design an answer key

Sometimes it is believed that writing open-ended questions is easier than multiple choice. That impression may be understandable given the large number of specific item construction rules for selected response items— which will be described in the next section in this chapter—but may not be that straightforward. Constructed-response questions require either a clearly defined answer key (in the case of short-answer questions) or a clearly defined set of requirements for a good response (in the case of longer constructed-response questions such as essays, theses, or other artefacts). Such an answer key or set of requirements also includes what is "out of scope"—that is, answers that might be encountered but are not correct or examples of artefacts that do not meet the requirements.

The construction of an answer key or clear definition of requirements is helpful for two reasons. First, these help the item writer check for clarity of questions; is the purpose of the question clear, are there any ambiguities with respect to wording, length, and level of detail of the question? Second, it will enable independent review by another assessor if so needed. Such answer keys or lists of requirements should therefore not be retrofitted.

Use only when the format is needed to assess the intended stimulus

This somewhat enigmatic advice means that constructed-response formats should not be used when things are being asked that could be easily and more efficiently asked with selected response items. For example:

— *Describe the numbers of lobes in both lungs.*

This can also be asked in a multiple-choice format.

Lungs are divided into several lobes. Which of the following options describes the numbers of lobes in both lungs correctly?

A. *Both lungs have two lobes.*
B. *The right lung has three lobes, and the left lung has two lobes.*
C. *The left lung has three lobes, and the right lung has two lobes.*
D. *Both lungs have three lobes.*

So, as a general rule, it is advisable to use constructed-response formats for questions that really require spontaneous answers. Typically, these are questions where an evaluation, critical analysis, comparison, creative production, and so on is required. This means that a question that asks for an underling reason or rationale is not necessarily such a creative question. This is an often-encountered misconception—namely, that when a question asks "why?" it automatically tests higher-order cognitive skills. But most of the required replies to these why questions are just repetition of learned answers. For example:

— *Why are monoamine oxidase inhibitors not the first-line treatment in depressions?*

It is logical that students answering this question will not be creatively constructing the rationale behind the question when they answer it. They will have learned this from their textbooks and will reproduce this learned rationale on the test.

Selected response items

Selected response items include single-best-option multiple-choice items, multiple true–false items (MCQs in which more than one option can or should be selected), true–false questions, extended-matching items, and script-concordance test items.

In this section we will describe more specifically the suggestions around writing MCQs because these suggestions pertain to the other format as well. Extended-matching items and script-concordance test items differ from the straightforward MCQ by including cases or vignettes. In later sections, we will discuss the tips that are specifically relevant for vignette or case base items.

An MCQ often consists of a stem or vignette in which the context of the question is described. This is the content in which the question is based. The question itself is often called the *lead-in*. The options consist of the correct option (answer or key) and the incorrect options or distractors. Open-ended questions are the same without options.

Example item:		
Stem:	*Mrs. Johnson is a 74-year-old woman who presents with complaints of bronchopneumonia with fever, nausea, and vomiting. She has been diabetic for many decades, and her blood sugars have been poorly regulated.*	
Lead-in:	*What is the most probable cause?*	
Options:	*A*	*Haemophilus influenzae*
	B	*Klebsiella pneumoniae*
	C	*Pneumocystis carinii*
	D	*Staphylococcus aureus*
	E	*Streptococcus pneumoniae*
Key:	*E*	

Although all MCQs in a test often have the same number of options—typically four or five—this does not necessarily have to be the case. Although studies have demonstrated the slight advantage in reliability between five- and four-option MCQs after several hours of testing time, this does not outweigh the practical constraints in many medical situations. Consequently, a good argument can be made to vary the number of options with the number of realistic alternatives. Having a fixed number of options sometimes leads authors to include unrealistic alternatives that undermine the credibility of the examination. Moreover, these options do not contribute to the measurement characteristics of the item because they are eliminated by virtually all the students.

An example of this is:

What effect do tropicamide eye drops have on the pupil?

A. *Pupil dilation*
B. *Pupil constriction*
C. *No effect*

In this case, it is obvious that no realistic fourth option could be found.

When creating an MCQ, it is good to start by writing it as a short-answer, open-ended question. This forces the author to think carefully about the point of the question unhindered by the options.

The most important item-construction guidelines are the following.

Make sure all options address the same aspect

Students should not be required to compare apples with oranges. When authors need to write many questions, they sometimes unintentionally add distractors that could be correct from a different viewpoint. The example below illustrates an item where this might be the case:

London is:

A. *A large city*
B. *Situated near the Atlantic Ocean*
C. *The capital of the United Kingdom*

Although option C is not absolutely correct (there are 29 places in the world with the name London) one can doubt whether A or B is true and whether London is nearer the Atlantic Ocean than it is a large city.

Generally, a so-called cover test is advised. This means that it should be possible to cover the options of an MCQ and still be able to answer it as if it were an open-ended question. If you were to cover the options here, the question would read "London is: . . . ." That is an unanswerable question. This construction rule is not trivial; research suggests that a proportion of the students prefer a so-called forward reasoning approach to MCQs, as if it were an open-ended question [23]. They will try to come up with the answer and only then look at the options. This forward reasoning has been associated with higher levels of expertise. So, making sure the question passes the cover test not only prevents unnecessary ambiguity but also allows students to use the forward reasoning approach.

Make sure all options are of similar length

As previously noted, ideally every item is a perfect predictor of the possession of knowledge or understanding, and so it should be written in a way that it is unlikely to lead to a false-positive response. Students will take advantage of item flaws, even if they do not know the correct answer. One of the simplest of these is to select the longest option. The longest option is more likely to be the correct answer because it typically takes more words to make an option defensively correct than to make it incorrect.

Make sure all options are of equal subtlety

Often options differ in level of subtlety. Real life is often much more nuanced than what can be presented in the stem or options. Consequently, the most subtle option is more likely to be the correct answer. The incorrect options generally do not need this level of subtlety and can be presented in a simpler and more direct way.

Make sure all options are worded in the same direction

It is unnecessarily confusing for candidates if some options are worded affirmatively but others are worded negatively. Combinations of positively and negatively worded options are likely to produce reading errors and lead to false-negative responses.

Test only one aspect per option

Two-in-one options not only make the item less clear; they also make it vulnerable to the so-called conversion strategy. Here is an example of two-in-one options:

> A patient has an arthritis of his left toe that developed spontaneously in a matter of 1–2 hours. His doctor suspects it might be a bout of gout. To determine whether this patient has gout an X-ray of the joint can be taken, a blood test for uric acid can be performed, or fluid can be drawn from the joint and examined.
>
> Which of the following options is correct concerning the sensitivity of these tests?
>
> A. X-ray higher than uric acid and higher than joint fluid examination
> B. X-ray lower than uric acid and lower than joint fluid examination
> C. X-ray lower than uric acid and higher than joint fluid examination
> D. X-ray equal to uric acid and higher than joint fluid examination

In the first comparison, the word *lower* is used twice; in the second comparison, *higher* is used twice. Option C contains the combination of both most-frequent comparisons and is therefore more likely to be correct. This is again logical because typically the author starts with the correct option and then varies on it. Another, less conspicuous example is the following:

What is the upper limit of normal AST in a healthy adult?

A. *< 4.8 U/l*
B. *< 48 U/l*
C. *< 60 U/l*
D. *< 480 U/l*

This example is less obvious, but the conversion strategy also works here. The options A, B, and D are all variations on 48, so they form a cluster of the numerals 4 and 8. The options B and C are of the same magnitude and so form a cluster as well. By applying the conversion rule, option B must be the correct answer. Two-in-one options can be used if they cover all possible combinations. In our first example, the problem would have been solved by a change of the fourth option into:

A. *X-ray higher to uric acid and higher than joint fluid examination*

A frequent example of the two-in-one problem is when each option contains a possible answer and an addition qualifying statement—typically a reason why the option would be true. This is illustrated in the following example:

A group of researchers wants to compare the effectiveness of a new e-learning module on pharmacodynamics to the traditional approach of lectures and practicals. They employ a typical causal comparative research design with a pretest to establish baseline knowledge and differences between the intervention and control group and a posttest to determine the differential effects of the interventions. The number of participants in each intervention arm is 50.

Which of the following is the most appropriate statistical analysis in this case?

A. *Separate Mann-Whitney tests because the scores are not normally distributed.*
B. *A two-way ANOVA because the number of participants in each group is high enough to use parametric statistics.*
C. *Separate chi-square tests because it is necessary to establish the association between the intervention and the outcome.*
D. *A Kruskall-Wallis test because statistical normality of the variable can be assumed.*

These questions are typically written under the assumption that students will have to think harder to better understand why an option is correct or incorrect. Unfortunately, this is not the case. The more information in an option, the more cues will be given. So, although there is more information in each option, it actually makes the question easier.

Make sure to word the questions clearly and unambiguously

Although we have discussed clarity in the section on constructed-response items, it pertains to selected response items as well. If all the items are intended to be individual small *diagnostic tests* for the absence or presence of knowledge or competence, it is also important to minimize false-negative results (students answering the question incorrectly despite having sufficient knowledge). Text that is difficult to read and understand may lead students to answer the question incorrectly because they did not understand it well enough. One could, of course, expect academic students to be able to read and understand more complex text, but if they answer a question incorrectly because of reading errors it is not a test of their knowledge. So, it is advisable to avoid unnecessarily complicated sentences. Sometimes, in an attempt to reduce the word count of an item, ambiguity is produced. As a rule of thumb, it is better to use more words and be clearer than to use fewer and be more ambiguous.

The options should cover the whole range of realistic options wherever possible but no more than the whole range

Covering the whole range of realistic options may be difficult, especially when the number of options is fixed and limited, but it still important to try to be as complete as possible.

For example, this question does not cover all options:

The sensitivity of a standard chest X-ray for the detection of tuberculosis is:

A. *greater than 90%*
B. *smaller than 75%*

The option "between 75% and 90%" is not included, so students who thought that the correct answer was between 75% and 90% know that their initial thinking was incorrect. The opposite is also problematic. If a subset of the options already covers the whole range of possibilities, the additional options are useless, for example:

Administration of propanolol in the majority of the cases leads to:

A. *a decrease in blood pressure*
B. *an increase in blood pressure*
C. *no measurable changes in blood pressure*
D. *a delayed response in blood pressure changes*
E. *few side effects*

For the test-savvy student, D and E do not have to be considered because A, B, and C have covered all realistic possibilities; the drug either increases or decreases the mean blood pressure or has no influence. There is no situation imaginable in which options A, B, and C are all incorrect. Students who consider this have just increased their probability of a successful guess from 0.20 to 0.33

Make sure the options are mutually exclusive

If there is overlap between the options, students are given a powerful cue to strategically eliminate incorrect options. For example:

The overall likelihood of developing mesothelioma after exposure to asbestos lies:

A. *between 0 and 10%*
B. *between 10% and 30%*
C. *between 20% and 40%*
D. *between 30% and 50%*
E. *between 40% and 60%*

Any percentage between 20% and 50% makes two options correct. For example, if students thought it was between 20% and 30%, they would have to choose between options B and C—and both would be correct. If they thought it was between 30% and 40%, options C and D would be correct, and so on. Therefore, the student now knows that it is either less than 20% or more than 50% and just has to choose between options A and E.

Make sure that only one option is defensibly correct—and that all the other options are defensibly incorrect

This is especially important if it is a single-best-option MCQ. Sometimes item writers focus on making sure that the correct option is defensibly correct but forget to check that the other options are completely incorrect. In such cases it can be helpful to formulate the lead-in specifically in that way; for example, "Which of the following is the *most* likely diagnosis?" rather than "Which of the following is the correct diagnosis?" This lead-in also allows for the author to test the use of judgment, and it is more consistent with clinical realities.

Avoid using collective options such as "all of the above" or "none of the above"

Research clearly shows that the use of collective options has a negative impact on the validity of the measurement of knowledge and understanding [24]. This is easiest to understand in the case of an "all-of-the-above" option. Suppose there are five options—four with a unique content and one collective. With those items, every student who knows at least two of the other options are true can automatically conclude that option E must be correct. You could ask a question in which more than one option is correct (the so-called multiple true–false items), but in a standard single-best-option MCQ it is best not to use collective options.

For the opposite, it is easy for a candidate to answer the item correctly based on incorrect information. For example:

In which province of the Netherlands is Amsterdam located?

A. *South Holland*
B. *Friesland*
C. *Limburg*
D. *None of the above*

Those candidates who think that Amsterdam lies in any of the other eight Dutch provinces will also respond with D and produce false-positive responses. Amsterdam lies in the province North Holland. So, ideally the question would have as many options as there are provinces in the Netherlands.

Check your items for grammatical cues, especially misalignment between lead-in and options

For students, it is crucially important to pass the examination, so they will use any information at their disposal to come up with the correct answer. Consider the following question:

Ipratropium is used in the treatment of asthma. It is an:

A. *anticholinergic*
B. *beta-2-sympahtomimetic*
C. *corticosteroid*
D. *xanthine derivative*

Because only option A starts with a vowel and thus aligns with the article *an*, cunning readers can easily conclude that A is the correct option. The other options start with a consonant and therefore would have required the article *a*.

Do not provide logical cues

Apart from grammatical cues, there can also be logical cues. Logical cues are elements of the item that can be solved using common sense rather than medical knowledge as illustrated in this example:

A patient consults you because of radiating pain from his lower back to his left gluteal region and his left leg. The pain increases when he coughs or sneezes. There are no complaints of loss of sensitivity of a motor functions. All reflexes of the lower extremities are intact and symmetrical. The most indicated treatment is:

A. *NSAIDs for pain relief*
B. *physiotherapy*
C. *surgery*
D. *electromyography*
E. *MRI*

Of course, this is a bit of a caricature but certainly an easy item for most students: Options D and E are not realistic. They are not treatment options, so the students in this case only have to consider options A, B, and *C*.

Avoid providing too absolute or too open options

Every option that has "can," "is possible," or synonymous words are hard to defend as being incorrect. In medicine, there are always exceptions to rules, so it can always be defended that something is possible even if it is highly unlikely. On the other hand, options with overly absolute statements such as "always," "never," "pathognomonic," and so on are so absolute that they are rarely defensibly correct. If you really want to focus on something that "can" or "cannot," be sure to include a statement that clearly describes the context in which you are asking the question. For example, when asking a medicolegal question, include statements such as:

> *In disciplinary procedures there are certain measures judges can use in their ruling, and there are measures that he/ she cannot use. Which of the following measures can the judge use?*

Avoid using so-called semiquantitative terminology

Unfortunately, our textbooks and also many published scientific papers are replete with rather vague and semiquantitative terms (*often, seldom, frequently, usually*, etc.). However, this does not mean that they can easily be used in written items as well. It is not clear how often *often* is or how seldom *seldom* is. When reading books or scientific papers, this can often be inferred from the whole context, but that context is often not present in a question. When semiquantitative terms are used in isolation there is substantial variation in how people use them, especially if they are asked to express them as a percentage [25].

Place the options in either alphabetical or another logical order

We do not know exactly why, but especially with four-option MCQs, option C is more likely to be the correct option. We assume this has to do with the way item writers work. Choosing option A as the correct answer may be unattractive because it gives authors the feeling they are giving the answer away immediately. It is more likely that they seek a distractor for option A and then a second one for option B. Regularly finding three distractors is more difficult, so the item writer uses C as the correct answer, and it acts as a sort of placeholder while the author tries to come up with the third required distractor. This may not be true in all cases or even in many, but whatever the underlying explanations, students also know that C is more likely to be the correct answer. So, their motto is, "When you do not have a clue, go for option C." The remedy is simple; you either put the options in a logical order—such as increasing severity of disease, invasiveness of the procedures, and so on—or in alphabetical order.

Keep it simple

Often it is believed that when questions are made more complicated, they test understanding or insight better than straightforward MCQs. An example is a question in which two statements are presented with a conjunction and the student has to indicate for each statement whether it is true and whether the connection is true. Another example is a list of statements, with the options presenting combinations of these various statements; the student has to indicate which statements are correct. However, it is unlikely that such complicated formulations test higher-order cognitive skills. There is overwhelming evidence that the content of the question is far more important than its format with respect to what the question assesses [9,26]. A more important distinction is whether the question is case based or a straightforward factual knowledge-based question. So, keep the question format simple but focus on the content.

Do not be afraid to use more words to explain exactly what you mean

Although parsimony and succinctness are good, they should never come at the expense of clarity. We have already suggested using extra words if they are needed to ensure clarity. Often, item writers are concerned about the additional reading time. This is only a minor issue, though, because reading time is much less of a cognitive demand than doubt about what was intended with the question. Of course, we all know the funny examples on the Internet of students providing correct but completely unintended answers to open-ended questions such as, "Where was the Declaration of Independence signed?" with the answer "At the bottom of the page." The answer is correct, but it is clearly not what the question intended. Whereas this illustration is just funny, questions such as "Which veins empty into the right atrium?" could lead to the answer "All veins eventually do." Again, the student may be correct, but it is not what the question writer intended.

We realize that these are only a selection of the issues that can be considered for item review and that there might be many more, but we think these are the most important.

PATHWAYS OF ITEMS IN THE QUALITY ASSURANCE PROCESS

The early 1980s witnessed an interesting discussion in the literature about validity. Cronbach contended that validity was purely a matter of how the test scores behave [27]. He saw validity mainly as a characteristic of the test scores—for example, whether test scores adequately captured increasing levels of expertise, or whether a newly developed test would add unique information to what was already obtained with existing tests. In this view, individual items are not meaningful in themselves but only to the extent to which they contribute to a valid total score. This validity thinking was built largely on psychological testing. One of the famous psychological tests, the Minnesota Multiphasic Personality Inventory, contains items such as "I would try to get into the cinema without paying if I was sure I would not be caught." This item is not intended to be meaningful in itself and is not aimed at assessing the person's cinema entry behavior but it is intended to say something about aspects of the test taker's personality in conjunction with other items.

Another famous psychometrician, Robert Ebel [28], contended that educational tests were not the same as psychological personality tests. In the latter, it was defensible to include content that did not have to be meaningful in and of itself but it would in the former. The clash between these views can be especially observed in observation-based clinical skills examinations such as Objective Structured Clinical Examinations (OSCEs). In traditional OSCEs, station scores are combined to calculate an overall average score for *skills*. This means that poor performance on abdominal examination can be compensated by a good knee examination. The station's *abdominal examination* and *knee examination* do not stand alone but draw their meaning based on their contribution to the measurement of *skills*. To many practicing clinicians, this is quite counterintuitive.

However, the point that Ebel made—that items on a test need to be intrinsically meaningful—is important and forms the basis for much of our thinking about quality assurance in assessment and the role item review committees play in this process (see **Case 3-2**).

Case 3-2: Concerns with the Perceived Relevance of Assessment Items	
Things to Consider	**Response**
What was the identified problem/need in your program relative to assessment?	At a medical school there were repeated concerns with the perceived relevance of items on one of the major assessment instruments. Although the school claimed that the items of that test were attuned to graduate level and were aimed at functional and relevant knowledge, student complained that many items were too detailed or not relevant to be known by heart.
What is the specifically needed assessment?	It was suggested to install a relevance evaluation committee for each item, but it was soon realized that such a committee would not assist in creating more relevant items and would run the risk of creating an adversarial relationship between the item writers and staff involved in the quality assurance processes.
What did you create to address this need?	After extensive consultation with stakeholders a narrative rubric was constructed to facilitate conversations about relevance of items. This will be demonstrated below.
What assessment principles were employed?	The principle used here is that issues of quality of an item have to be discussed and that agreement, shared subjectivity, has to be reached. Attempts to quantify quality—apart from the obvious oxymoronic relationship between these words—would have led to adverse effects in the organization.
What were the outcomes/ lessons learned?	Creating and using agreed upon narratives to communicate and reach sufficient agreement on matters of item quality has led to better collaboration and understanding of each other's roles, when the rubric was used actual relevance (for example as indicated by psychometric properties of items) was more predictable and in item review committees it was very helpful in improving the quality of items.

Item review committees

It is fair to say that items that are not reviewed before they are used in an examination are much more likely to have item-construction flaws than items that have been reviewed [29]. Here we repeat that, ideally, each item is a small diagnostic test for the absence or presence of knowledge or competence. The item review is focused on minimizing the likelihood of false-positive and false-negative results. Therefore, many organizations and universities have panels that critically review draft questions and provide the item writer with suggestions for improvement.

Organizationally, these meetings can be positioned differently in the process of producing examinations. The most common arrangement is one in which the draft questions are collected long before the examination will be administered and reviewed by the panel. Such an organizational structure has an advantage because the purpose of the review panel is clearly visible. The purpose is then defined as helping to produce *this* examination.

There are other ways to organize quality assurance, however. For example, in an ongoing process, items can be produced on a regular basis by the teaching staff. This may take place when they are triggered to write an item—for example, when they are teaching or working clinically, while they are doing their own literature search, or when they encounter common misconceptions or relevant points for learning. These questions are then collected in a pool. The review panel meets on a regular basis to review the items in the pool. After they have been given the okay, they are moved into an item bank from which questions can be drawn for future examinations. Figure 3-1 shows both designs.

It may be clear that for such processes the inclusion of an item bank is indispensable. However, it is also clear that the item bank is not built to automatically draw examinations but to assist in managing the quality assurance process. This is an important point; too often organizations invest into designing or buying expensive item banking systems under the assumption that the systems will allow them to automatically generate examinations. This often leads to disappointment. An examination is more than just a random selection of questions; questions may become outdated rather quickly or at least must be updated, and automatically generated examinations may have unwanted overlap between questions. More importantly, to ensure the integrity of the information that would be required to automatically generate examinations, the amount of work that needs to be put into the item bank may surpass the amount of work saved. So here, too, the keep-it-simple principle applies, and it is probably more efficient to use the item bank to support the production and quality assurance process. With respect to supporting the production process, automated item banks

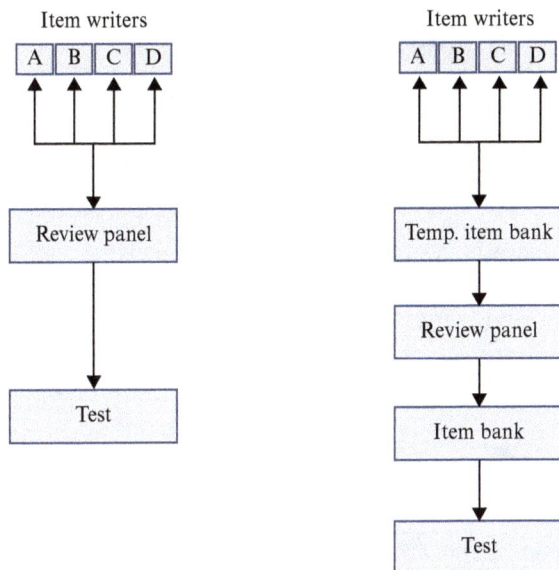

Figure 3-1 • Single-cycle quality assurance processes.

can be useful in generating overviews of how many items on each topic or domain are available so that item writing can be more targeted.

The two schemes in Figure 3-1 are based on a quality-control process that uses only one cycle: quality assurance before the test administration. However, a second cycle of quality control can be added. A second review process can follow the test administration. Typically, psychometric information, so-called item analyses, can be reviewed. In addition to that, student comments and critiques can be incorporated. This quality assurance cycle can lead to items being withdrawn from the test, answer keys being changed, or items even being eliminated from the item bank because of fundamental flaws. Figure 3-2 shows possible arrangements of such a quality assurance cycle.

Review panels, composition

An appropriate mix of staff members with sufficient knowledge of the subject matter to understand the questions and answers are best positioned to be members of review panels. They need to be able to critically question content, phrasing, and relevance of items. Of course, superspecialists may be excellent at judging the content, but they may lose sight of what is relevant, for example, for a normal medical graduate. Because they are so well versed in the subject matter, they may also overlook some issues with phrasing because they take implicit meanings for granted. Having an open conversation, attempting to construct

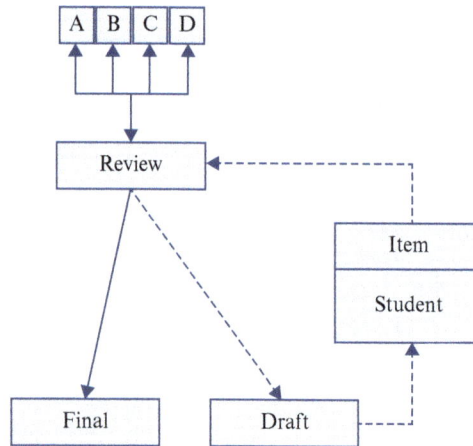

Figure 3-2 • Dual cycle quality assurance processes.

arguments for the relevance of each item may be helpful (see Table 3-1). Consequently, diversity in professional backgrounds is useful. A combination of basic scientists with clinicians in review panels or even in combination with behavioral scientists is also helpful. It is extremely important and relevant to the role of the chair of the committee to create a culture in which "not knowing" can be safely expressed. The expertise of all committee members is limited, and no one has expertise on all domains of medicine. We all have things we know and things we do not. If it is impossible to create a culture in which this "not knowing" is acceptable, then critical concerns about questions will not be voiced. If this is the case, review committee meetings are less useful [30].

Item review is a process that requires high-level logistical and administrative support to coordinate the review panel's activities, maintain the item bank, and ensure proper version control of items. Without proper support, even the best review panels in the world may be incapable of producing high-quality test papers (see **Case 3-3**).

Item review committees that change the items without conferring with the original author may appear to be efficient but run the risk of turning the review committee into a "foreign body." It should always be clear that the item writer has content knowledge about the item and that the role of committee members is to support the item writer in producing the best possible question. So, in an ideal situation, every examination question is a co-construction between the item writer and the review panel. It must never be a discussion about power or righteousness but a collaboration. So, when providing authors feedback, it is important to acknowledge that item writing is always difficult, especially when a staff member has to write many items. Making an error is not an indication of lack of expertise, it is often just an oversight and we all have our own blind spots. Therefore, the following four elements are ideally present in the feedback:

1. What is the incorrect aspect of the question? What is the content problem—is it concern with the formulation or the relevance that has caused the panel to flag the item? When it concerns standard item-construction flaws, it is best to use standard feedback such as that given in the previous sections.
2. Explain why this is a problem. You may, for example, use the false-positive and false-negative response concept to explain how the item-construction issue may lead to a false-positive or false-negative response. You may also indicate how it is likely that particular flaws would lead to random results (as is the case for example with "all of the above" and "none of the above" options).
3. If possible, present solutions as to how the question could best be rephrased or changed to mitigate or even eliminate the flaw. In our experience, giving concrete suggestions for revision with the explanation most often gets the item writer on board and agreeable to the proposed solution.
4. Finally, it is important to indicate how and why you think the suggestion for revision makes a better question than the original version.

The feedback to the item writers on formulation can be done using the suggestions in item writing in this chapter. It is also good to be critical about content of the item. Different well-established sources do not always agree and—as said before—good items need to be such that a correct answer is defensibly correct, and the others are defensibly incorrect. The most difficult issue to provide feedback on though might be relevance.

Table 3-1 EXAMPLE OF AN ARGUMENTATION TABLE FOR RELEVANCE OF ITEMS		
Extent to which the knowledge has to be readily available		
The knowledge can be easily and quickly found; even specialists do not need to have this readily available.	The knowledge can be relatively easily found, but it is convenient in practice (also for speed) if the graduate has it readily available.	The knowledge has to be readily available; it is obvious 2 AM knowledge because it either cannot be found quickly and easily or the medical situation may not allow the time or affordances to look it up.

(continued)

Table 3-1   EXAMPLE OF AN ARGUMENTATION TABLE FOR RELEVANCE OF ITEMS

Appearance in the curriculum

This aspect is rarely mentioned in the curriculum. It is knowledge that is not needed as a foundation to understand other more complex concepts.	The knowledge in itself may not be relevant, but it is a foundation to understand other concepts (Bohr-Haldane effect to understand why hemoglobin releases oxygen in the tissues but absorbs it in the lungs).	This knowledge is repeatedly present in the curriculum or may form the basis for many different concepts and has to remain explicit in those concepts (for instance to be able to explain to patients) (e.g., Frank-Starling mechanism as basis for heart failure, medication, etc.).

Relationship with practice

No practical situation can be found in which this knowledge is explicitly needed.	There are practical situations thinkable, but they are clearly farfetched and unlikely to occur, be encountered by a graduate, or do not need to be managed.	It is easy to find multiple practical situations in which this aspect has to be explicitly known and used.

Practical relevance

This is rarely encountered in practice; it is generally rare or something only relevant in highly specialized centers.	It is knowledge in the context of prevalent or medium- to high-risk practical situations, but the explicit knowledge is not necessary for the successful management of such situations.	It is knowledge in the context of prevalent or medium- to high-risk practical situations, and the explicit knowledge is necessary for the successful management of such situations.

Specific knowledge for medicine

It is not specifically medical knowledge; a layperson would know this as well.	It is not specifically medical knowledge, but a layperson would be able to acquire this knowledge with a bit of searching.	It is specific medical knowledge, and a layperson would not be able to acquire this knowledge with a bit of searching; it requires deep study and understand of other aspects of medicine as well.

Case 3-3: Lessons Learned through the Development of Post-test Quality Assurance Procedures

Things to Consider	Response
What was the identified problem/ need in your program relative to assessment?	A Regulatory Body conducts written multiple choice examinations for licensing of international medical graduates in examination centers throughout the world. Great care is taken in the quality assurance of assessment material before the examination
What is the specifically needed assessment?	However, there were few to no post-test administration quality assurance, and given the high stakes of the examination and its outcomes this additional cycle of quality control was absolutely necessary.
What did you create to address this need?	Two kinds of data are considered. Incident reports on venues are compiled by venue staff. They deal with issues such as physical and space issues, candidate welfare and potential security breaches or compromises. A comprehensive statistical report is also presented to the Panel. Overall examination statistics are compared to those of previous examinations and individual items are calibrated. Each examination contains pilot or trial items. Their performance is analyzed, and recommendations made about their inclusion in future examinations. Separate analyses are also conducted for item performance by examination venue and country of training as well as performance in patient groups or disciplines. The latter are represented in the examination through selection of items according to a carefully-developed blueprint. Discipline leaders on the Panel communicate information on item and examination performance back to their respective writing groups for revision of both existing and new pilot items.
What assessment principles were employed?	The principles of dual quality control cycles, diversity of information sources and member checking were included
What were the outcomes/ lessons learned?	The combination of all quality control processes has improved the corporate knowledge and expertise on examination development, delivery logistics and has been the instigator for several research and development process.

Another good moment to give feedback to item writers is after the test has been administered and analyzed. Often, item writers are experts in their field, and they may find it difficult to gauge the appropriate level of difficulty of an item. Item writers who teach regularly and have close contact with their students might be better at it, but feedback on item performance helps them better align the difficulties of their items with the levels of their students.

Another opportunity for providing feedback is to inform members of standard-setting panels. There are numerous—around 40—different methods described in the literature [31]. Regardless of the method, they are all based on judgment on what is reasonable. So-called absolute standards typically use the judgment of experts about what is reasonable to expect from a borderline candidate or group of candidates. Standard-setting methods such as those from Angoff and Ebel require panels of experts to judge the difficulty of each item for that specific group of candidates (for an overview, please see [32,33]). There are compromise methods such as that from Hofstee that require decisions about acceptable pass–fail levels and acceptable pass–fail percentages [34]. Even so-called norm-referenced methods use assumptions and judgments about what can be reasonably expected of the candidates. In general, judgments become better if they are better informed, and feedback on the actual performance of the students and of the items (item analyses) is therefore an important way to ensure that judgments in the standard-setting process become better informed.

▌ ITEM ANALYSES

In previous sections we alluded to the process of item analysis several times. These are item-specific statistics that can be calculated after the test administration and used for quality control. Typically, item analyses give an impression about how a group of students performs on a particular test. So, item analyses usually provide a picture of the qualities of the items in relation to a group of test takers.

For example, if an item is answered correctly only by 10% of the students (it has a so-called p value of 0.10), it could mean that the item is flawed or difficult. Alternatively, it could signify that the students did not work hard enough and did not master this topic. A third possibility is that the students were not being taught well. In medical education, large groups of students are typically quite stable in their level of competence, so an item with a low p value is more likely an issue with the teaching, motivation, or the item case itself rather than the student cohort's average competency. The conclusion could be that it has to be given more attention in the course or the way it is taught must better align with the learning capacity of the students.

The consequence of poor item statistics is always a matter of judgment, and there should always be a further investigation to understand why an item performed poorly. We argue that in the vast majority of the cases it is not a good idea to eliminate an item merely based on its item statistics. In research, we do not eliminate data because we do not like the statistics unless a clear analysis has shown that the data were indeed invalid. The same applies to assessment; if item analyses show abnormal outcomes, further investigation should determine whether the question was indeed valid (correct content, correct formulation, and relevant part of the examination) before it is removed.

Item analysis parameters

Often used parameters are:

p value

This is the proportion of students who answered the question correctly. A p value of 1.00 means that all students have answered the item correctly. If the p value is 0.00, none of the students has answered the question correctly. For a competence-orientated test, you may want to accept any p value as long as the item is relevant for the topic and has been taught in the course. For example, for a test that seeks to support decisions about entry into medical school, you may want to have p values that are not too close to either 1.00 or 0.00 because they do not add to the discrimination between the students about whom you wish to make judgments. As a rule of thumb, ranges between 0.25 and 0.75 (0.30–0.70) are often used. It is commonly thought there must be something wrong with a question when the p value is lower than the chance score. For example, in a MCQ with four options, one can argue that *on average* there is a 25% chance of a correct answer and therefore the p value should not be lower than 0.25. This is a misconception, however; the chance score is *on average*—that is, across multiple items—and this does not mean it has to be 0.25 for each item.

a values

Used predominantly in MCQs, an a-value signifies the portion of students who chose an option from among the other options in the question. The a value of the correct option is the same as the p value. Again, their interpretation is based on the purpose of the test. In a test for selection, the distractors (false options) need to be attractive for those who do not know the answer. If they are not, the question does not contribute to the distinctions among candidates. If the test is competence orientated or in an educational context, it is less important if a distractor is unattractive, as long as it indicates that the students know that this is not the right answer (and not, for example, because the distractor was so poorly worded that the student could guess it wasn't the right answer).

q-values

Q values are 1 minus the p value; they indicate the proportion of students who answered the question incorrectly.

R_{it} or item-total correlation (or discrimination/point-biserial) and R_{ir} or item-test correlation

The R_{it} is the correlation between the item and the total score on the test. In other words, the R_{it} indicates whether the question was predominantly answered correctly by those students who also had a high score on the test and not by those who had a low test score. It is an indication of the extent to which the item contributes to the total test score (cf the discussion between Cronbach and Ebel previously mentioned). Because the R_{it} is a correlation, it is a value between -1.00 and $+1.00$. The value of $+1.00$ means that the item perfectly correlates with the rest of the items and contributes maximally to the total score, and a value of -1.00 means that the item contributes negatively to the total score. In other words, the item was answered correctly by the students who had the lowest scores on the total test and incorrectly by those who had the highest scores and test. There is an alternative to the R_{it}: the R_{ir} or item-test correlation.

On examinations with small numbers of items—for example, a 10-item short answer question examination—the total score is influenced by the item itself because it constitutes one-tenth of the total score. If the item total correlation (R_{it}) were used here, there would be a problem of autocorrelation, and the item performance would be correlated with at least 10% of the total score. That typically spuriously increases the item-total correlation. So, the R_{ir} is an alternative and it is the correlation between the item and the score on the rest of the items. The point-biserial correlation is another way of describing this relationship. It is worth mentioning again that these values are highly dependent on the cohort of students and the other items on the test. Also, the values will be different, depending on what metric is used (how the correlations are calculated). So be careful not to over interpret the values always ask more questions about how they were calculated and then go back to the items and see what these statistics can tell you. They are only there to inform your judgment.

CONCLUSION

Quality assurance processes of written assessment are essentially focused on ensuring that each item or assignment is a sensitive and specific diagnostic test for the presence of knowledge, insight, understanding, and so on. Therefore, an item must be optimally clear; when student misconceive the meaning or purpose of the item, they cannot provide a response that will be validly and reliably interpreted. This chapter has provided an explanation of what contributes to quality, guidelines for the construction of high-quality items and assessment, examples and tips around the design of quality assurance procedures during the production stage of the assessment, and, finally, quality assurance processes after assessment delivery. This chapter is by no means complete, there are numerous handbooks and published articles for this, but it has hopefully provided a sufficiently comprehensive overview.

REFERENCES

1. Cilliers FJ, Schuwirth LWT, Adendorff HJ, Herman N, Van der Vleuten CPM. The Mechanisms of Impact of Summative Assessment on Medical Students' Learning. *Advances in Health Sciences Education.* 2010;15:695–715.
2. Cilliers FJ, Schuwirth LWT, Herman N, Adendorff HJ, Van der Vleuten CPM. A Model of the Pre-Assessment Learning Effects of Summative Assessment in Medical Education. *Advances in Health Sciences Education.* 2012;17:39-53.
3. Gielen S, Dochy F, Dierick S. Evaluating the Consequential Validity of New Modes of Assessment: The Influences of Assessment on Learning, Including Pre-, Post- and True Assessment Effects. In: Segers M, Dochy F, Cascallar E, eds. *Optimising New Modes of Assessment: In Search of Qualities and Standards.* Dordrecht: Kluwer Academic Publishers; 2003:37–4.
4. Shepard L. The Role of Assessment in a Learning Culture. *Educational Researcher.* 2009;29(7):4–14.
5. Schuwirth LWT, Van der Vleuten CPM. Programmatic Assessment: From Assessment of Learning to Assessment for Learning. *Medical Teacher.* 2011;33(6):478–485.
6. Albanese MA, Mejicano G, Mullan P, Kokotailo P, Gruppen L. Defining Characteristics of Educational Competencies. *Medical Education.* 2008;42(3):248–255.
7. Young M, Thomas A, Gordon D, et al. The Terminology of Clinical Reasoning in Health Professions Education: Implications and Considerations. *Medical Teacher.* 2019:1–8.
8. Kane MT. Validation. In: Brennan RL, ed. *Educational Measurement.* Vol 1. Westport: ACE/Praeger; 2006:17–64.
9. Ward WC. A Comparison of Free-Response and Multiple-Choice Forms of Verbal Aptitude Tests. *Applied Psychological Measurement.* 1982;6(1):1–11.

10. West R, Farrow S. A Comparison of Different Examination Marking Systems for Medical Students. *Medical Teacher*. 1996;18(3):241.

11. Anbar M. Comparing Assessments of Students' Knowledge by Computerized Open-Ended and Multiple-Choice Tests. *Academic Medicine*. 1991;66(7):420–422.

12. Durning SJ, Dong T, Ratcliffe T, et al. Comparing Open-Book and Closed-Book Examinations: A Systematic Review. *Academic Medicine*. 2016;91(4):583–599.

13. Schuwirth LWT, Van der Vleuten CPM, Donkers HHLM. A Closer Look at Cueing Effects in Multiple-Choice Questions. *Medical Education*. 1996;30:44–49.

14. Schuwirth LWT, Verheggen MM, Van der Vleuten CPM, Boshuizen HPA, Dinant GJ. Do Short Cases Elicit Different Thinking Processes Than Factual Knowledge Questions Do? *Medical Education*. 2001;35(4):348–356.

15. Sales D, Sturrock A, Boursicot K, Dacre J. Blueprinting for Clinical Performance Deficiencies—Lessons and Principles from the General Medical Council's Fitness to Practise Procedures. *Medical Teacher*. 2010;32(3):e111–e114.

16. Schmidt HG, Norman GR, Boshuizen HPA. A Cognitive Perspective on Medical Expertise: Theory and Implications. *Academic Medicine*. 1990;65(10):611–622.

17. Boshuizen H, Schmidt HG. On the Role of Biomedical Knowledge in Clinical Reasoning by Experts; Intermediates and Novices. *Cognitive Science*. 1992;16:153–184.

18. Case SM, Swanson DB. Extended-Matching Items: A Practical Alternative to Free Response Questions. *Teaching and Learning in Medicine*. 1993;5(2): 107–115.

19. Bordage G. An alternative approach to PMP's: the "key-features" concept. In: Hart IR, Harden R, eds. *Further Developments in Assessing Clinical Competence: Proceedings of the Second Ottawa Conference*. Montreal: Can-Heal Publications Inc; 1987:59–75.

20. Ebel RL. *Essentials of Educational Measurement*. Englewood Cliffs, NJ: Prentice-Hall; 1972.

21. Miller GE. Continuous Assessment. *Medical Education*. 1976;10:81–86.

22. Case SM, Swanson DB. Constructing Written Test Questions for the Basic and Clinical Sciences (https://www.nbme.org/publications/). 1996. http://www.nbme.org/publications/item-writing-manual-download.html

23. Maguire TO, Skakun EN, Triska OH. Student Thought Processes Evoked by Multiple Choice and Constructed Response Items. In: Scherpbier A, Van der Vleuten C, Rethans J, et al., eds. *Advances in Medical Education: Proceedings of the Seventh Ottawa Conference on Medical Education*. Dordrecht, The Netherlands: Kluwer Academic Publishers; 1997:618–621.

24. Harasym PH, Leong EJ, Violato C, Brant R, Lorscheider FL. Cueing Effect of "All of the Above" on the Reliability and Validity of Multiple-Choice Test Items. *Evaluation and the Health Professions*. 1998;21(1):120–133.

25. Hakel MD. How Often Is Often? *American Psychologist*. 1968;23(7):533–534.

26. Norman GR, Smith EKM, Powles AC, et al. Factors Underlying Performance on Written Tests of Knowledge. *Medical Education*. 1987;21:297–304.

27. Cronbach LJ. What Price Simplicity? *Educational Measurement: Issues and Practice*. 1983;2(2):11–12.

28. Ebel RL. The Practical Validation of Tests of Ability. *Educational Measurement: Issues and Practice*. 1983;2(2):7–10.

29. Downing SM, Haladyna TM. Test Item Development: Validity Evidence from Quality Assurance Procedures. *Applied Measurement in Education*. 1997;10(1):61–82.

30. Verhoeven BH, Verwijnen GM, Scherpbier AJJA, Schuwirth LWT, Van der Vleuten CPM. Quality Assurance in Test Construction: The Approach of a Multidisciplinary Central Test Committee. *Education for Health*. 1999;12(1):49–60.

31. Cusimano MD. Standard Setting in Medical Education. *Acad Med*. 1996; 71(10 Suppl):S112–120.

32. Livingston SA, Zieky MJ. *Passing Scores: A Manual for Setting Standards of Performance on Educational and Occupational Tests*. Princeton NJ: Educational Testing Service; 1982.

33. Berk RA. A Consumer's Guide to Setting Performance Standards on Criterion-Referenced Tests. *Review of Educational Research*. 1986;56(1):137–172.

34. Hofstee WKB. The Case for Compromise in Educational Selection and Grading. In: Anderson SB, Helmick JS, eds. *On Educational Testing*. San-Francisco, CA: Josey-Bass; 1983:109–127.

4 Quality Assurance of Objective Structured Clinical Examinations

Katharine Boursicot, Sandra Kemp, and Richard Fuller

CHAPTER HIGHLIGHTS

- Quality assurance is important to ensure fair, robust, and defensible outcomes.
- Application of the Kane Validity Framework as a quality assurance tool
- Objective Structured Clinical Examinations (OSCEs) and the COVID-19 pandemic

▌ ORIENTATION TO THE CHAPTER

Objective Structured Clinical Examinations (OSCEs) are widely used to assess clinical, communication, and practical skills in medical education, especially in high-stakes contexts. The quality assurance of an OSCE is therefore of critical importance to ensure that such tests are fair, robust, and defensible. OSCEs are highly complex to design and implement, and many different aspects have to be scrutinized. We have taken a specific approach to quality assuring OSCEs, using what we refer to as the Kane Validity Framework, because this provides a holistic and systematic framework to use when evaluating the quality of an OSCE. This chapter begins by setting the context of OSCEs within a learning and competence taxonomy, then moves onto describing the features of the Kane Validity Framework. The next section of the chapter describes the application of each section of the Kane Validity Framework in relation to OSCEs. Templates are provided for use when working through the different aspects of quality assuring OSCEs. Other quality assurance mechanisms and issues are described, including the special circumstances that the COVID-19 pandemic has placed on the conduct of OSCEs, at the time of writing. The chapter concludes with a summary of how quality assurance of OSCEs should be conducted in a systematic and holistic manner to ensure that defensibility, credibility, and fairness are maintained and signposts show opportunities for further assessment enhancement.

INTRODUCTION

Within a frequently used learning and competence taxonomy that is applied to clinical competence [1], OSCEs align with the "shows how" level of clinical competence in Miller's pyramid. (See Figure 4-1.) As such, OSCEs are an assessment method fit for purpose when assessing a student's or trainee's (or a candidate's) ability to perform particular clinical skills. As a consequence, OSCEs are currently regarded as the best format for integrated, high-stakes summative assessment of clinical competence using a single test format. OSCEs typically assess across a range of clinical skill domains—for example, physical examination, consultation and communication skills such as consent, clinical reasoning, and technical or procedural skills [2].

Although there is extensive literature about OSCEs, there is limited work that provides practical advice on how to quality assure an OSCE. When approaching quality assurance of an OSCE, several factors should be scrutinized in a systematic manner so that evaluation of the quality of the test or examination in terms of validity, reliability, and fairness is a consistent and coherent exercise. This more holistic approach has evolved from a narrow focus (and arguably misinterpretation) of the usefulness

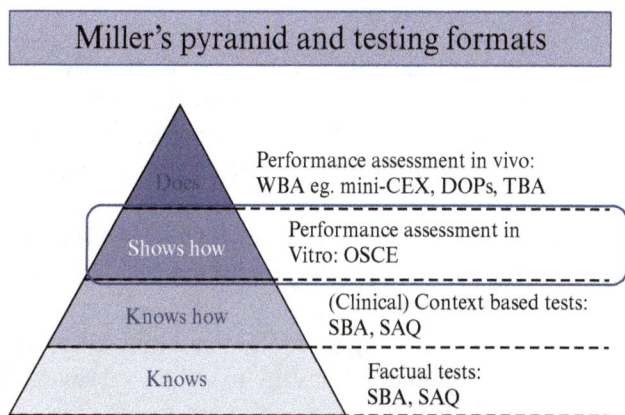

Figure 4-1 • The Place of OSCEs in Miller's Pyramid of Clinical Competence [1].

of psychometric parameters as the sole measures of assessment quality. Further, some approaches to the quality assurance of OSCEs have been inconsistent and unsystematic, leading to claims about competence that are not supported by evidence.

This chapter focuses on the quality indicators related to OSCEs and does not address other assessment formats that were previously common for assessing clinical skills. For a review of these formats, see the Ottawa Consensus Statement on Performance Assessment [3] and the AMEE Guide to OSCEs (Part 1) [4].

Assessment of clinical competence is complex and inference based, so we describe the application known as the Kane Validity Framework [5] as a theoretical framework to use in quality assuring OSCEs. This focuses on contemporary approaches to quality assurance that have moved from a previously dominant psychometric view to a broader approach that requires defining the purpose for using the test results and the collection of relevant evidence to support the justification of the uses of the test results [6]. This inference-based approach to validity [7] allows the collection and analysis of a wider range of evidence sources compared to other validity approaches (e.g., unitary validity [8]) and is ideally suited to the OSCE, which assembles policies, processes, measurements, and outcomes as sources of evidence in order to make a judgment about defensibility.

QUALITY ASSURANCE USING THE KANE VALIDITY FRAMEWORK

The Kane Validity Framework is a holistic and comprehensive approach to evaluating assessment quality that is gaining increasing recognition and use in the medical education world [9–12]. The outputs from this validity-based approach are multipurpose, affording both quality assurance of assessment (a requisite for institutional, regulatory, candidate, public, and other stakeholder confidence) and quality improvement (understanding where OSCEs may need further development such as station design or examiner training).

The Kane Validity Framework involves three sections or phases. The first involves defining the intended purpose of the test. The second relates to gathering relevant evidence to support the intended use of the test. This includes aspects such as planning of content, internal structure, response process, consequences, and relationship to other variables. The third refers to the justification for the use of the test results. We discuss each phase in turn to explain quality assurance processes and decisions related to OSCEs.

Phase One—Defining the Intended Purpose of the OSCE

Following the Kane Validity Framework, the first quality assurance task is to look for a clear *purpose statement*. This should be a distinct statement about what the OSCE is supposed to be testing and, if applicable, where it fits within the system of assessment for that program, course, or post-graduate training pathway. Arguably, a good assessment system should have an overarching purpose, with definable purpose statements for each supporting component or test, such as the OSCE.

First, there should be clarity about why the OSCE has been chosen as the testing format. OSCEs were originally designed for and remain most appropriate for testing clinical, communication, and practical skills in a more controlled, clearly structured context (an examination situation) where the candidate demonstrates an aspect of clinical performance and an observer views and scores the performance [2]. If the tasks required to be performed by the candidates in an OSCE do not involve the demonstration of clinical skills, then this raises serious questions in relation to validity evidence and fitness for purpose.

Second, be transparent about how the OSCE results will be used. For example, a statement might indicate that the results will be used to make a decision about whether a candidate is able to progress from one stage of a program to the next, graduate, or be awarded a specialist degree. A good example of a set of purpose statements can be found on the website of the UK Royal College of General Practitioners in relation to its membership examinations [13].

Phase Two—Gathering Relevant Evidence to Support the Intended Use of the OSCE

The second phase of applying the Kane Validity Framework relates to how different types of evidence can be gathered to support the intended use of the test. The following five aspects are important to focus on from a quality assurance perspective. Each will be discussed in turn:

1. Planning of content
2. Internal structure
3. Response process
4. Consequences
5. Relationship to other variables

Planning of content

An important part of quality assurance is inspecting how an OSCE's content is planned. In preregistration medical education contexts, how they become part of a system of assessment is important for quality assurance, although this may not be applicable for other medical and health professions contexts. Where an OSCE is part of an assessment system, there should be information about how it fits in the overall system of assessment [14,15], with other information about how knowledge and application of knowledge are tested, how Workplace Based Assessment (WBA) is used, longitudinal approaches to professionalism assessment [16], and how all assessments (including the OSCEs) are deployed over the course or program. See Figure 4-2 for an example of a system of assessment.

In addition to situating the OSCE with the range of assessments mapped to the overall curriculum (when part of an assessment system), there should be appropriate content alignment for the OSCE itself. As such, there should be a blueprint of the OSCE that details the domains of competence being tested and demonstrates mapping to the learning objectives or outcomes of the relevant part of the course or program.

Designing a *system of assessment*: aligning assessment to learning outcomes—themes, domains and tools

Curriculum themes and graduate outcomes	Scientific foundations of dentistry	Patient and dentist: clinical practice	Professional and personal development
Domain of competence	Knowledge and application of knowledge	Clinical and communication skills	Professional practice
Assessment tools	Single best answer (SBA)	OSCEs	• Professionalism tools • WBAs • Discursive writing
Year 1 Year 2 Year 3 Year 4 Year 5	• Formative written tests (SBAs) • End-of-year paper: 240–300 SBAs	• Formative OSCEs • End-of-year OSCE: 14–18 stations	• Professionalism assessment • WBAs • Projects or essay • Research

Figure 4-2 • Example of a System of Assessment across an Undergraduate Dental Program.

System	History Taking	Explanation Negotiation	Examination	Practical Procedures
Number of stations	5	3	5	7
Cardiovascular	Chest pain		Cardiac	BP
Respiratory	Hemoptysis		Respiratory	Peak flow
Gastrointestinal	Abdo pain		Abdomen	PR
Neurology	Loss of consciousness	Anti-epileptic compliance	Sensory legs	Fundoscopy
Musculoskeletal			Hip	
Urology				Catheter insertion
Endocrine	Palpitations	Diagnosis of DM (1)		
Generic		Consent for postmortem		Set up IV
				Phlebotomy

Figure 4-3 • Example of an OSCE Blueprint for a Graduation Level OSCE for a Pre-registration Medical Program.

The blueprint should also describe how many stations are planned with an appropriate rationale. See Figure 4-3 for an example of an OSCE blueprint.

Quality review steps for blueprinting include review and consensus building by stakeholders to analyze the coverage of the blueprint. Important questions for stakeholders to consider (and documentation of same) include: Are the required systems or disciplines covered by this individual OSCE? Is the spread across different systems or disciplines adequate? Is there balance between the domains reflecting the stage of training? There should also be evidence of faculty content and expert agreement that the chosen cases represent population demographics and evidence must be documented that expert clinical faculty have created and reviewed the cases and scoring schemes. Accompanying the visualization of alignment (blueprint) is a clear statement of the *rules* that determine the construction of the OSCE (test specification). This will clearly set out the decision rules around the number, type, and duration of stations, often further mapped to key domains (e.g., a certain number of prescribing skills stations or a certain number of stations related to a body system such as the respiratory system).

Where there are multiple OSCEs within a system of assessment, quality review steps that adopt a longitudinal lens are required. Important questions for reviewers to address include:

- Are the required systems or disciplines sampled appropriately across time, and are any inappropriate emphases across multiple stages avoided?
- Are different presentations and underlying conditions blueprinted across the different stages of training (and any repetition is deliberately by design)?
- Does the sampling reflect the types of expected or planned learning experiences that OSCE candidates have had?
- Is there scaffolded progression from models or manikins to simulated patients to actual patients across time as appropriate to each skill domain? Effectively, are we showing the added value of stations in senior years of training, with an intentional approach to aligning expected experience?

Internal structure

An important aspect of quality assurance relates to *internal structure*, and this includes important information about how the OSCE is designed (including number and length of stations), individual station design, aspects of examiner training, what the scoring scheme is, how the pass mark is set and the measurement and interpretation of post hoc psychometric analyses of the OSCE results.

One of the most critical elements of using OSCEs is sufficient sampling. If there are too few stations, the OSCE not only will have low reliability but also will be unlikely to provide a relevant breath of assessment of key curriculum content [17]. The length of stations (time the candidate spends in the station performing the skill) should be stated. Different tasks may require different timings, so timing is determined as appropriate to the task. This information should be addressed in the blueprint or test specification.

Scoring Schemes: Scoring or marking schemes typically use either a checklist or a rating scale. Originally, checklists were universally used in OSCEs, but research over the last 20 years has shown that rating scales demonstrate better validity and interrater reliability than checklists [18]. With rating scales, examiners can determine not only if a task was done or not (as in a binary checklist item) but also how well the task was performed. More recently, reconceptualization of checklists as nonbinary formats, the importance of score design, and alignment with the clinical task being assessed have demonstrated that checklists can be effectively utilized [19,20]. This highlights the importance of selecting a scoring format that is appropriate for the task being undertaken or examined, the level of the candidate, and arguably the experience of the examiner pool.

Domain-based rating scales are a way of constructing a scoring schedule for OSCEs that enables qualitative descriptions of dimensions of quality performance to guide the scoring process. The domains follow the classic steps of a doctor–patient interaction: approach to the patient, taking a history, clinical examination, planning investigations, and management. A review of the quality of domain-based marking schemes should be planned as a regular activity in consultation with users of the marking scheme, clinical experts, and education experts with experience in rubric design. Review of quality needs to consider the aspects such as relevant domains for the task, descriptors and language used, and rating labels. Descriptors need to be appropriate for the stage of training. Table 4-1 lists the areas to guide a quality review as well as key aspects that should be critiqued.

An example of one skill domain (physical examination) from a domain-based rating scale is provided in Table 4-2. This illustrates five distinct levels of performance, using qualitative descriptions.

Irrespective of format used, scoring should be designed to align to the tasks or behaviors expected to be measured in each OSCE station and learning outcomes being assessed. For checklist formats, it is helpful to follow the sequence of the task being performed (e.g., checklists can be of greater use in procedural type stations where clinical practitioners will often internalize a checklist-type approach to safe practice). For domain-based marking schemes, it is useful to follow the phases of the consultation being observed. Quality assurance should be demonstrated by a review of the scoring format (and examiner instructions) by appropriately qualified faculty.

Standard Setting and Psychometric Analyses: Standard-setting methods and psychometric analysis of OSCE data form a critical part of quality assurance of internal structure. Although detailed discussion of standard-setting methods is outside the scope of this chapter, it is important to note that, especially if the OSCE is a high-stakes one, the standard-setting method should be a criterion-referenced (absolute) one rather than a relative method or an arbitrary score [21,22]. Whatever method is used, there should a rationale described for the choice of method based on best practice from the literature. The choice of approach will depend on the design of the OSCE and particularly the number of candidates and context of the assessment.

Table 4-1. DOMAIN-BASED MARKING SCHEME QUALITY REVIEW

	Quality Review	Key Aspects to Critique
1	Are the relevant domains included in the appropriate station type?	Are all components of history taking accounted for as a whole? Do all the history-taking stations have the same set of domains? Are key areas such as professionalism and patient input included in every station?
2	Does each descriptor for each standard for each domain contain a qualitative (not quantitative) description?	Each descriptor needs to qualitatively describe the performance. For example, what does a "competent" performance look like in that domain? Are numbers and counting avoided?
3	Does each descriptor reflect the ways clinicians think about performance in that domain?	Is the language used reflective of how clinicians would describe good or poor clinical performance?
4	Does each descriptor clearly delineate the difference between one level of performance and the next?	Are there clear and distinct descriptions of how one level of performance can be judged to be different from another level of performance? In other words, can the examiner, using the descriptor, clearly decide between a "competent" performance and a "not yet competent" performance?
5	Are the labels for the descriptors for the domain-marking scheme different to the overall rating labels used for borderline regression standard setting?	Do the labels enable examiners to make a conceptual shift between (a) a skill level in a particular domain such as communication (labels such as "acceptable" and "poor") and (b) making a judgment about the overall performance in the station such as "clear pass" and "borderline"?

Whilst a number of standard setting methods have been described in the literature, borderline methods—specifically borderline groups (BGM) and borderline regression (BRM)—have emerged as the "gold standard" in larger scale OSCEs with more than 100 candidates [22]. In both methods, decision-making is anchored around the expected performance of the "just passing" (or borderline) candidate and the use of larger scale data to generate a "cut point" or passing score that helps determine the station pass mark.

Table 4-2 SAMPLE OF DESCRIPTORS FOR PHYSICAL EXAMINATION DOMAIN

Domain	Outstanding	Competent	Acceptable	Poor	Very Poor
Clinical skills: physical examination	Performed all examination steps correctly and in the correct sequence. Examination was conducted smoothly and with fluency.	Performed all examination steps correctly and in the correct sequence.	Performed all examination steps correctly and in the correct sequence or small changes in sequence were not problematic.	Performed examination steps sometimes incorrectly or not in the correct sequence.	Limited evidence of correct steps or correct sequence.

This requires conceptualization and consensus on the performance characteristics of clearly satisfactory, unsatisfactory, and just passing performance relevant to the candidate cohort. Examiner training and clear articulation of these descriptors are essential parts of examiner support in OSCEs.

In both methods, examiners award score performance on the relevant in-station tasks (checklist, domain, hybrid scoring). With the BGM, candidates are also given an overall grade (fail, borderline, pass) based on overall performance in the station; the score distribution of only those candidates in the borderline group is examined in detail to determine a station-level passing score. With the BRM, typically five overall grades (e.g., ranging from unsatisfactory, just pass, clear pass and good pass to excellent) and all examiner-candidate scores and grades are plotted into a scatter graph and regression equations applied to determine the station-level cut score at the borderline. Unlike the BGM, the BRM approach uses all data from examiners and candidates to improve determination of the passing score [23].

These approaches can be undertaken via directly automated software (e.g., where institutions use smart devices to capture scores in an OSCE) or through simple applications in Excel or SPSS. Once station-level scores have been calculated, they are summed across all stations to provide an overall pass mark. To improve the granularity of decision-making, institutions may choose to apply an additional *conjunctive* standard (i.e., one that reuses the data from the exam) such as a requirement to pass a minimum number of stations outright in addition to the pass score or the addition of a standard error of measurement to the overall passing score [24].

Both approaches have relied on large enough groups of cohorts to provide a distribution of candidates across the unsatisfactory and borderline grades, mindful that in any cohort we should expect a skewed performance to pass (or better). Earlier work had suggested that a minimum of 50–100 candidates was required for borderline methods to be applicable; for smaller OSCEs, the use of the Angoff method remained most appropriate [25].

A recent paper has explored the impact of borderline methods in small cohorts in more detail, looking at three groups: (1) small cohorts in a physician associate training program, (2) sequential OSCEs, and (3) an international registration exam [24]. In all three cases, numbers of candidates were typically small (e.g., $n < 30$) and relied on either Angoff-derived station-level cut scores or extant data (where stations had been used previously in larger-scale exams). This work suggested more stability of the BRM than anticipated, primarily because of good station design and a wide ability spread of candidates and the use of global grade distribution. The key message from the body of work around standard setting echoes the need to choose a standard-setting method that is credible, defensible, and appropriate to the design of the OSCE and candidate cohort [26].

Following completion of the OSCE, post hoc psychometric analysis should be undertaken as key evidence in this validity-based approach to quality. It is essential that the analysis and interpretation is undertaken with full knowledge of the OSCE design and delivery phases, allowing informed decisions to be made about the choice of psychometric parameters and their interpretation. For multisite OSCEs or those with multiple circuits or cycles, more detailed analysis is required (e.g., to demonstrate no significant differences in overall SCORES achieved by candidates taking the OSCE at the end or start of the day or by site). It is critical to ensure that for these psychometric analyses to be of use, candidates must be randomly allocated to groups, circuits, and cycles. (Note that OSCEs with small numbers of candidates using Angoff methods for standard setting may yield more limited psychometric analysis.)

Typically, psychometric analyses produce two types of evidence: (1) about the OSCE as a whole (reliability) and (2) the stations within the OSCE using a "family" of station-level metrics akin to a suite of complementary diagnostic tests in clinical practice [27]. Overall whole-test reliability (internal consistency and reproducibility) provides some quality evidence that allows interpretation at the level of the cohort taking the test but less evidence to support individual pass–fail decisions. The use of reliability alone as a psychometric indicator is no longer recommended. It is also critical to ensure that an appropriate method of determining reliability is evidenced given the established limitations of Cronbach's alpha as a reliability measure for some OSCEs. See Figures 4-4a and 4-4b for examples of whole-test metrics.

Number of candidates	56
Number of stations	10
Cronbach's alpha	0.65
Average score	87.4%
Passing score	77.0%
SEM (Standard Error of Measurement)	2.3%
Pass rate	98.2% (55/56)

Figure 4-4a • Example of Basic Whole-Test OSCE Metrics.

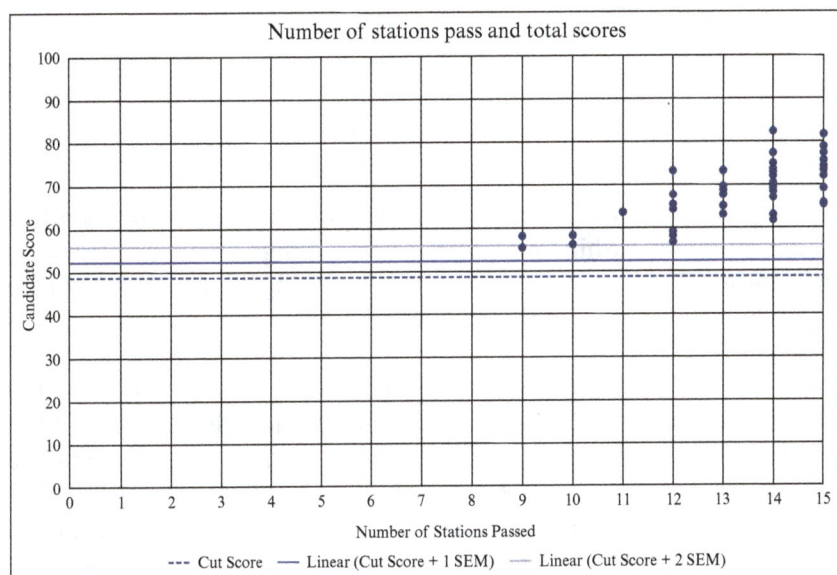

Figure 4-4b • Example of Basic Whole-Test OSCE Metrics.

At the station level, simple analyses can include the number of candidates passing or failing a station and the effect on the reliability coefficient if the station is removed (see Figure 4-5 for an example). This can also be useful longitudinally (across multiple diets of OSCEs using stations from a bank) to determine whether standards are changing [28]. Pell et al. describe a series of seven metrics specific to OSCEs that offer more information on station performance, relationships between checklist and global scores (especially when using the borderline regression method for standard setting) as well as looking at differences across OSCE circuits [29]. These analyses are critical to evidencing how stations "perform"

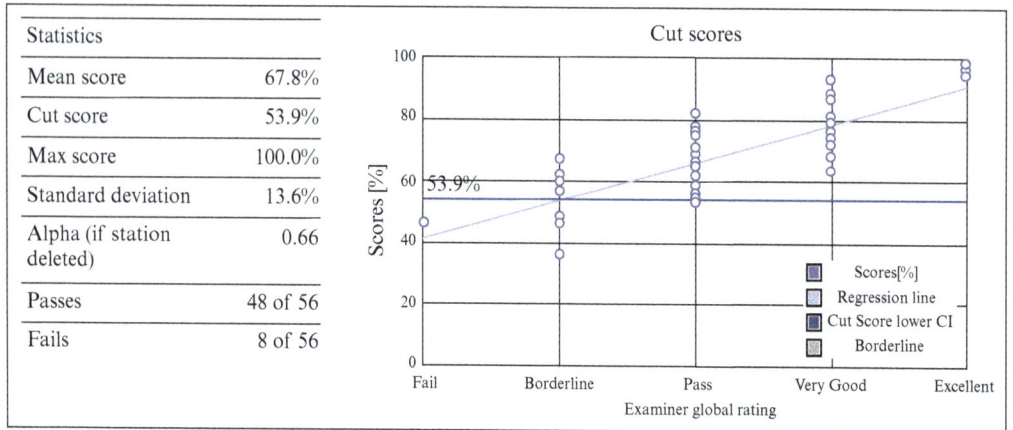

Statistics	
Mean score	67.8%
Cut score	53.9%
Max score	100.0%
Standard deviation	13.6%
Alpha (if station deleted)	0.66
Passes	48 of 56
Fails	8 of 56

Figure 4-5 • Example of Station-Level Metrics.

in any particular OSCE, and they can support a deeper understanding of the interrelationships of OSCE station design, examiner training, and scoring [30,31]. As indicated at the beginning of this chapter, these methods can also support OSCE quality improvement, as well as assurance [32].

Establishing a tracking process to quality assure the pass–fail decision-making for OSCEs is important. Where a high-stakes OSCE involves progression of the OSCE candidate to the next phase or stage of education, performance measures can be correlated to investigate how well progression decisions align with success in the next stage of education. Borderline passing candidates who subsequently underperform in the next stage of education may be an indication of pass–fail decision-making requiring a change.

Response process

Attention should be paid to how the OSCE is delivered in terms of ensuring fairness for the candidates. This would include aspects such as consistency of simulated patient (SP) role playing, examiner conduct, timing, equipment, access to venue, and how accurate collection of scores is ensured. This is especially important if more than one circuit is conducted and multiple sites are used. There are also considerations about test security. OSCE delivery is a major logistical undertaking that requires careful planning of circuit layout, signposting, and enabling candidates to clearly understand the instructions for the tasks to be undertaken at each station. Attention should be paid to SP training because variable performance of roles by the SPs will result in a variable experience for each candidate. Evidence should be sought about the effectiveness of the SP training program.

Examiner conduct can be a major destabilizing factor in OSCEs. This does not mean we expect examiners to be "standardized," and this is not a realistic outcome. However, as a minimum, examiners should have been briefed on the nature and purpose of the OSCE, be familiarized with the scoring system (especially if delivered electronically such as on tablet devices), and be exposed to some practice of scoring sample performances of "candidates" (e.g., video recordings or simulated performances using actors) [33].

There should also be evidence that examiners are scoring candidates fairly and accurately. There needs to be evidence that candidate scores are collected, stored, and used with attention to the appropriate interpretation of these data, typically through demonstration of examiner training, on the OSCE day briefing, and post hoc psychometric analysis of station performance.

Test security is an ongoing debated issue, and there is a perception by candidates that sitting the test later in a schedule and knowing what is coming up affords an advantage, but there is only limited evidence supporting this view [34]. If the stations in an OSCE truly test clinical skills, which are developed over time by practice and experience, it is questionable whether knowing what is coming up in the next few hours or the next day would give the candidates sufficient time to improve their skills. It should be part of the quality assurance process to check if candidates are allocated randomly across sessions and to undertake routine analysis for any systematic variations [35].

Consequences

The consequences of any OSCE should be clarified and communicated in advance. If the OSCE is for formative purposes (i.e., assessment for learning), this should be transparent and unambiguous to the candidates, and the results should not be used to contribute to any final grades. If the OSCE is being used for summative purposes, then the consequences of passing or failing should be clear to the candidates. For high-stakes OSCEs, it is critical that the pass-fail decisions are robust and evidence based [22,36] and institutional mechanisms for review and appeal are clearly described. One consequence that should be analyzed is the educational impact on candidates and how their learning behaviors relate to practicing clinical and communication skills. This connects to consequences of the OSCE on learning and quality assuring feedback. First, it is essential to ensure that feedback is provided to all OSCE candidates. Second, the feedback must be useful and actionable for candidates. In the context of OSCEs, feedback can be distinguished as either of the score reporting type or narrative type.

Feedback: For quality assurance of score-reporting feedback, a review of the type of feedback provided and a check of how well it aligns with the purpose of the OSCE is required. To provide quality score-reporting type of feedback, the skill domain being assessed is the focus. For example, skill domains that constitute the marking scheme could include areas such as:

- history taking or clinical content, which is the ability to elicit main points of history and logically sequenced structure and so on;
- physical examination, or the ability to perform examination steps correctly and in correct sequence smoothly; and
- presentation of findings, or the ability to correctly report all important and relevant clinical findings in a well-structured and coherent summary.

There will be multiple skill domains in an OSCE domain-based marking scheme, and these will vary by station type—that is, all history taking stations would use the same set of skill domains in the marking scheme. Some skills domains are common to different types of stations. Score reporting can then provide a broad view of strength areas in a particular skill domain across a number of stations. This skill domain breakdown is especially useful for feedback to identify strengths and weaknesses. An example is provided in Figure 4-6.

For OSCEs, another aspect of quality that should be reviewed is whether or not score reporting presents information that compares a candidate to other candidates. This should be approached with great caution and reviewed against the key purpose of learning. If, for example, the OSCE is predominantly for formative purposes, then comparative feedback can be problematic and undermine learning. However, it may be that in high-stakes OSCEs, comparison with other candidates is warranted.

However, score reporting (numbers as percentages or raw marks) does not provide information to the candidate about *how* to improve. Therefore, if the OSCE is part of a wider assessment system such as in

Analysis Graph — Scoring Domains

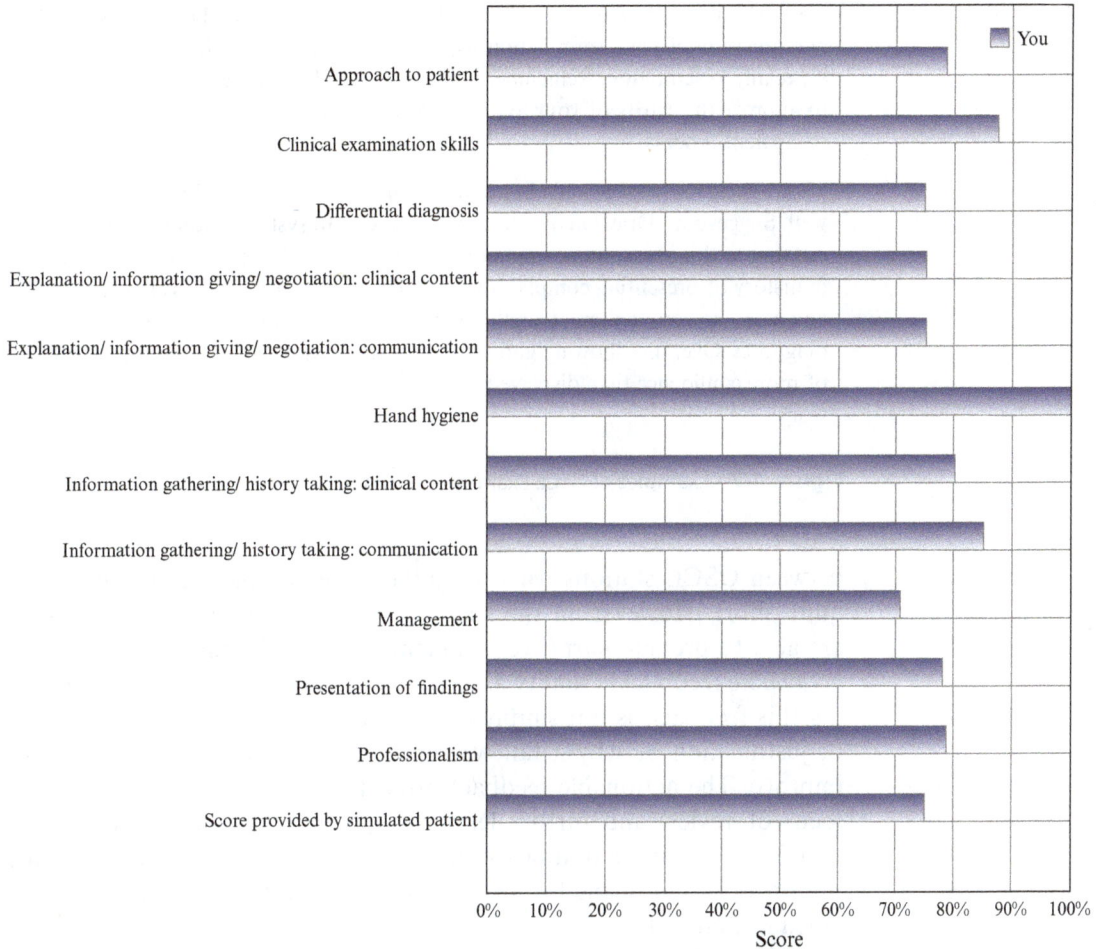

Figure 4-6 • Example of a Feedback Chart for Performance in Different Domains for One Candidate Across 15 Stations.

preregistration medical education, then quality review of OSCE feedback should check that narrative feedback is provided to OSCE candidates in addition to score reporting. Narrative feedback can provide information to candidates beyond what needs to be improved, which is what the candidate can glean from score-reporting feedback. Thus, candidates need to receive actionable feedback, and this is best provided during the OSCE by the observing OSCE examiner for each station. Typically, the time

Feedback comments for candidate (include at least one actionable comment

A sound examination process with appropriate patient manner. In future, keep working on your confidence and ease of communication as well as the flow and precision of your examination sequence. Be exact with each maneuver, especially auscultation. Remember to direct the medical feedback to the examiner to improve the clarity of your feedback. Keep at it as you have the basics of a competent process.

Shows good knowledge and clinical reasoning which is steering history taking well. Suggestion: Draw on questions you know from systems enquiry that are relevant to this presenting complaint (in this case breathlessness) and ask them in history of presenting complaint to round out the history (in this case resp and cvs)—so you don't miss anything (like palpitations). Ran out of time for diagnoses. Overall—showing good clinical history taking skills which are worthy of more confidence than displayed in the station—well done, keep up the good work!

Figure 4-7 • Examples of OSCE Examiner Feedback

between OSCE stations when examiners are completing the scoring is quite short. However, in the space of a couple of minutes, examiners are able to provide narrative comments and can be directed to provide *actionable* feedback. Quality assurance processes should focus on ensuring this feedback is not simply a description of what the candidate did or justification of why a fail was given but information about how to improve. The actionable feedback from the examiners can then be the focus of review and further learning. Quality assurance may indicate that further training in how to provide feedback may be required. Some examples of actionable feedback provided by OSCE examiners are provided in Figure 4-7.

Although feedback needs to focus on test takers, it is important that similar measures are evidenced to support examiner training and development at the level of the individual examiner (for new and experienced examiners) and in developing training packages (again for new examiners and "refresher" training for established examiners).

Relationship to other variables

The relationship between the OSCE scores and other variables, such as performance in other assessments, should form part of quality assurance processes for OSCEs. This is an often-neglected aspect of quality assurance in some sectors of medical and health professions education, but analyses that investigate these relationships can yield interesting and useful information. Comparing the OSCE results of candidates with knowledge tests is one possible approach, but looking at the performance of candidates in OSCEs compared with other clinical performance (such as national postgraduate examinations) could be more interesting and inform the usefulness of the preregistration medical education OSCEs [37]. Equally important is evidence indicating no correlation (or a strong negative correlation) with some other assessment that is hypothesized to be a measure of some completely different achievement or ability—for example, comparing the results of candidates on an OSCE with knowledge tests. The longitudinal monitoring of candidates as they progress through a program or system of assessment can often reveal key evidence about the strength of assessment and the progress or development of borderline or just passing candidates [38].

Triangulation of clinical skill performance in OSCE skills domains, with clinical skill performance in other performance assessments such as WBAs will provide additional information to inform quality review. This also aligns more with programmatic approaches to assessment [10].

Phase Three—Justification for the Use of OSCE Results

The final phase of the Kane Validity Framework is to construct an "argument" or justification for how the OSCE test results are used. This is a complex process and requires a summary and interpretation of all the validity evidence to form a justification. Therefore, this phase of the framework consolidates its previous two phases and would be part of a comprehensive monitoring and evaluation process.

Summary of Framework

The Kane Validity Framework is increasingly used in medical education as a framework to review and evaluate tests in a systematic manner [7,39–44]. It supports more synoptic or holistic approaches to assessment quality that is emerging in national assessments [45] and international standards of excellence in assessment [46]. When engaging in quality assurance, two critical questions must be asked:

1. Are the outcomes of the OSCE defensible?
2. Are the outcomes of the OSCE credible, fair, and transparent?

Using the Kane Validity Framework enables a systematic approach to answering these questions. This more comprehensive approach to test design and quality assurance focuses attention on a range of important specific elements of test design, construction, and delivery, going some way in redressing the overemphasis on a single source of evidence (such as reliability) as the only criterion for quality assurance. See **Appendix 4-1** for an example of a workbook for an OSCE applying the Kane Validity Framework, which provides a step-by-step approach to the first two sections of the framework. Prompts guide the user in each step.

Once an OSCE is scrutinized using the Kane Validity Framework, an OSCE Quality Improvement Report can be generated. It is important to document quality improvements made as a part of quality assurance. See **Appendix 4-2** for an example that includes some samples of how this might be achieved. Clear documents such as this template can ensure that processes and outcomes are documented and transparent to different stakeholders.

OTHER QUALITY ASSURANCE MECHANISMS AND ISSUES

The Kane Validity Framework provides a useful lens through which to quality assure. Remember: Applying the framework enables this holistic quality assurance evaluation, but this does not equate to justifying the practice of referring to it as a *validated test*. A test should not be referred to as *validated* as if this was a stamp of permanent quality; a test is only valid for the particular context in which it was designed and used. Transferring a test for use in a different context does not guarantee validity, and the quality assurance framework should be applied to the test in its new context.

In some countries, established processes are common and may not use a framework, instead being more process oriented. For example, and as already highlighted in **Chapters 1** and **2**, the external examiner process is common in some countries such as the United Kingdom.

External Examiner System

The external examiner system is where professional colleagues in a similar institution are invited to review examinations. Please note the term *external examiner* is used to refer to an individual who observes the OSCE process, not a station-level examiner or assessor who is external to the institution that is conducting the OSCE. Ideally, it would be an individual who has assessment knowledge and skills, and this might be combined with clinical content expertise. In some circumstances, assessment expertise might be provided by one individual and content expertise provided by another. It can be useful to provide guidance about the core areas that an external reviewer or external examiner should scrutinize and provide feedback on as part of evaluating your OSCE. See **Appendix 4-3:** External reviewer/ examiner report for OSCE. Many countries also have other collaborative processes functioning as an alternative to an external examiner system to review and share as part of quality improvement and quality assurance.

OSCEs in a Pandemic Context

COVID-19 is a coronavirus infection that spread across the world from late 2019 to pandemic proportions through 2020 and into 2021. Apart from the public health issues, COVID-19 has presented significant challenges for medical schools, both for clinical placements and disruptions to clinical or performance assessments that require face-to-face contact with patients, such as OSCEs. Please see **Chapters 7** and **10** for further discussions on the impact of COVID-19 on assessment within the medical education context.

The response to keep participants safe has been varied: from cancellation of all clinical examinations to a variety of "remote" OSCEs. (We use the term *remote OSCEs* to refer to an OSCE that is conducted through all or many participants in a virtual environment). However, many of the reported "adaptations" have deviated and are misaligned from the fundamental principles of assessment of clinical skills through an OSCE [47–49]; that is, candidates are required to demonstrate performance of a clinical task and should be observed in that performance to make a judgment of competence [2]. The main challenge has been testing physical examination skills and practical skills, with only a few examples reported [50,51].

The pandemic may have long-term effects on how clinical workplaces are managed, and this is likely to have an impact on OSCE design and implementation. For example, infection risk is minimized through restrictions on mixing patients, candidates, teachers, and examiners across sites. The most fundamental consideration from a quality assurance and assessment perspective is ensuring that clinical skills across different domains are assessed, and some skills can only be demonstrated in the presence of a patient or simulated patient. Some of the solutions developed to deliver OSCEs during the COVID-19 pandemic could well be adapted into routine practice, reflecting not just novel ways in which technology might be used for OSCE delivery (technology enhanced learning and assessment) but also reflecting authentic clinical practice (technology-enabled health care). The increasing use of video technology to conduct remote patient consultation, an increasing approach to *device-augmented health care* (e.g., bedside ultrasound scanning) or the use of cloud-based data services to remotely connect and integrate radiology and laboratory information during the consult provide exciting opportunities for the OSCE to keep pace with the world of work and may become routine in the future [52].

▌ CONCLUSION

Quality assurance of an OSCE involves a complex array of aspects that need to be planned in advance, analyzed systematically, and reported. Evaluation of the quality of an OSCE is always in terms of validity, reliability, fairness, transparency, and using consistent and coherent processes underpinned by evidence from the literature. We have provided a framework that can be used to inform and guide the quality assurance processes. The Kane Validity Framework is our interpretation of the complexity associated with defining the purpose of the OSCE, gathering relevant evidence to support the OSCE's intended use, and the justification of the use of the OSCE results. The use of this type of framework ensures a systematic approach to quality assurance and can replace or complement existing quality mechanisms. Referral to a framework such as this will ensure that in ever-changing or unpredictable circumstances, it is possible to successfully design and implement quality OSCEs and have defensible decision-making for the outcomes of OSCEs.

In conclusion, quality assurance of the OSCE is detailed, complex, and essential to ensure decisions about pass–fail protect learners, institutions, and patients most of all. Increasingly, the use of more holistic approaches such as contemporary validity theory allow the assembly of complex data from multiple sources to examine and ensure defensibility of the test scores from the OSCE and their use. However, these approaches also underpin the quality improvement of the OSCE. It is now more than 40 years since the OSCE was first described, and the design, content, and scope of clinical performance assessments has continued to evolve to align with contemporary clinical practice. The "deep-dive" approach that validity requires identifies key opportunities for institutions to continue to develop new, innovative clinical performance stations through better understanding of design, candidate and examiner issues, intelligent use of standard setting and psychometrics, and, most importantly, developing more actionable feedback for candidates, examiners, and testing institutions.

APPENDIX 4-1: VALIDITY FRAMEWORK: WORKBOOK FOR AN OSCE

The following **Validity Framework** is to guide the stages of OSCE design and development

SECTION 1	**INTENDED USE OF THE OSCE** This section relates to: **1)** the purpose of the OSCE **2)** the intended use of the OSCE **3)** who the intended users of the OSCE are, both OSCE test takers and users of OSCE results
SECTION 2	**EVIDENCE TO SUPPORT THE INTENDED USE OF THE OSCE** This section relates to: • how the content of the OSCE is decided • how you design OSCE stations/circuit, at test level • how the OSCE is administered and conducted • how the consequences of the OSCE are managed

▌ SECTION 1: INTENDED USE OF THE OSCE

No.	TASK	QUESTIONS
1.1	Explain the main purpose/s of this OSCE	• Why is this assessment important to conduct as a part of your system of assessment? • How does this OSCE fit into the assessment system as a whole? (i.e. relationships to other OSCEs and other assessments) • Why should students/trainees complete the OSCE? • What key skills do you expect students/trainees to demonstrate? • How is the timing of your assessment important? • How does this OSCE connect with teaching/education/curriculum?
1.2	Explain the intended use/s of the OSCE	• Will the OSCE scores be norm-referenced or criterion referenced? • What are the stakes associated with the OSCE scores? (i.e. progression, licensing, etc.)

(Continued)

No.	TASK	QUESTIONS
1.3	Explain who is taking the OSCE and who will be using the OSCE results	• Who is the OSCE designed for? • How diverse are the OSCE test takers? • Are there characteristics of the OSCE test takers that should be taken into account? • Who is the audience for the OSCE results? Who uses the results and what do they do with the results?

WRITE A PURPOSE AND INTENDED USE STATEMENT
(summarize the answers to the questions in section 1 into one statement)

SECTION 2: EVIDENCE TO SUPPORT THE INTENDED USE OF THE OSCE

SECTION 2A: Planning of content

No.	TASK	QUESTIONS
2A	Explain how the OSCE has been blueprinted	• How will key skills be sampled in the OSCE: History taking, physical examinations, professional encounters (such as explaining) and procedures/practical skills? • How is the sampling mapped to the learning objectives/outcomes/competencies? • How will you ensure the OSCE tasks align with the OSCE test takers stage of education/training?

CREATE THE OSCE BLUEPRINT
(a matrix with clinical skills domains (e.g., history taking, physical examination, professional encounter and procedures) on X axis and curriculum domains (e.g., systems/disciplines) on Y axis)

SECTION 2B: Internal Structure

No.	TASK	QUESTIONS
2B	Explain how the OSCE is structured	• How many stations are planned? • How long is each station? • What are the marking/scoring schemes in each station? • What is the plan for circuits?

CREATE THE OSCE PLANS
(draw circuit design, write marking schemes, write station information sheets, SP scripts, reasonable adjustments plan, etc.)

SECTION 2C: Response Process (Administration and conduct of the OSCE)

No.	TASK	QUESTIONS
2C	Explain the mechanisms for scoring	• Is the assessment scored electronically or on paper? What are your safeguards in relation to recording the student score accurately? • What are the safeguards for recording and auditing for any changes to student scores?

DOCUMENT THE SECURITY AND AUDIT TRAIL PROTOCOLS

SECTION 2D: Consequences of the OSCE

No.	TASK	QUESTIONS
2D 1	Explain the standard setting methods used	• What standard setting method will be used to determine the passing standard? • What are the passing criteria? Do a minimum number of stations need to be passed? Are there other compensation/noncompensation rules, or weighting rules applied? • How is the Standard Error of Measurement used for determining the final passing score?
2D 2	Explain the impact on stakeholders of the OSCE	• How do you report scores and feedback to OSCE test takers • How do you report scores to educators/supervisors/public? • How do you manage the impact on test takers if they fail the OSCE? • What arrangements are there for resitting/remediation/support? • Is there any feedback loop from the OSCE results, to the curriculum/teaching/education? • Is there any feedback loop to the OSCE planners and administrators?

DOCUMENT THE STANDARD SETTING METHODS, PASSING CRITERIA, AND REPORTING ON THE OSCE

APPENDIX 4-2: OSCE QUALITY IMPROVEMENT REPORT

OSCE Quality Improvement Report	
Quality Improvement Aspect	**Response**
What is the purpose that underpins the use of an OSCE?	• Summative test of individual students' clinical and communication skills to pass to next stage of program of study (graduation)
What was the identified problem or need in your assessment program related to the OSCE?	• Poorly designed summative OSCE: assumed, not stated purpose • No blueprint, arbitrary pass mark, stations inconsistent in design and scoring, insufficient sampling, no feedback • Unfair and indefensible; students passing who did not have appropriate skills/competencies
What measures did you take to address this need?	• OSCE blueprinted: test content mapped to the stated learning objectives of the relevant part of the course • Scoring schedules modified • Criterion-referenced standard setting introduced • Feedback for students implemented • Engagement of faculty to design better stations • Examiner training and calibration introduced • Better information for students about OSCE process
What review principles were employed?	• Kane Validity Framework • Feedback from examiners • External reviewer engaged
What were the outcomes?	• Improved test design, including better metrics • Rating scales preferred by examiners; more engagement • Robust standard setting: better credibility, better feedback for students who needed to improve

APPENDIX 4-3: EXTERNAL REVIEWER, EXAMINER REPORT FOR OSCE

OSCE being observed:

- Institution
- Level
- Site
- Date

Name of External Reviewer/Examiner:
Affiliated institution:
Position in Institution:

Date of report:

Level of Examination

Did the level of the OSCE match similar levels of student examinations in your institution?

General Aspects of the Examination

- Blueprinting: Did you consider the examination blueprint appropriate?
- Standard setting: pass–fail determination process
- Logistics of the examination
- Examiner briefing
- Examiner conduct
- SP conduct
- Student briefings

Stations

History-Taking Stations

- Were the cases appropriate?
- Were the cases reflective of local demographics and disease prevalence?
- Was the time allowed adequate for the assigned task?
- Any specific comments regarding a station?
- Scoring scheme: How well did the scoring assess the students" performance?

Clinical Examination Stations

- Were the cases appropriate?
- Were the cases reflective of local demographics and disease prevalence?
- Was the time allowed adequate for the assigned task?
- Any specific comments regarding a station?
- Scoring scheme: How well did the scoring assess the students" performance?

Explanation and Negotiation Stations

- Were the cases appropriate?
- Were the cases reflective of local demographics and disease prevalence?
- Was the time allowed adequate for the assigned task?
- Any specific comments regarding a station?
- Scoring scheme: How well did the scoring assess the students" performance?

Practical Skills Stations

- Were the cases or tasks appropriate?
- Was the time allowed adequate for the assigned task?
- Any specific comments regarding a station?
- Scoring scheme: How well did the scoring assess the students" performance?

Overall Impression

Other comments

(observations and recommendations for improvements)

▋ REFERENCES

1. Miller GE. The Assessment of Clinical Skills/Competence/Performance. *Academic Medicine*. 1990;65(9):S63–S67.
2. Kogan JR, Conforti L, Bernabeo E, Iobst W, Holmboe E. Opening the Black Box of Clinical Skills Assessment via Observation: A Conceptual Model. *Medical Education*. 2011;45(10):1048–1060.
3. Boursicot K, Etheridge L, Setna Z, et al. Performance in Assessment: Consensus Statement and Recommendations from the Ottawa Conference. *Medical Teacher*. 2011;33(5):370–383.

4. Khan KZ, Ramachandran S, Gaunt K, Pushkar P. The Objective Structured Clinical Examination (OSCE): Part I: An Historical and Theoretical Perspective—AMEE Guide No. 81. *Medical Teacher*. 2013;35(9):e1437–1446.

5. Kane MT. Validating the Interpretations and Uses of Test Scores. *Journal of Educational Measurement*. 2013;50(1):1–73.

6. Downing SM. Validity: On the Meaningful Interpretation of Assessment Data. *Medical Education*. 2003;37(9):830–837.

7. Cook DA, Brydges R, Ginsburg S, Hatala R. A Contemporary Approach to Validity Arguments: A Practical Guide to Kane's Framework. *Medical Education*. 2015;49(6):560–575.

8. Messick S. Validity. In: Linn RL, ed. *Educational Measurement*. New York, NY: Macmillan; 1989.

9. Lineberry M. Validity and Quality. In: Yudkowsky R, Park YS, Downing SM, eds. *Assessment in Health Professions Education*. London, UK: Routledge; 2020:17–32.

10. Schuwirth LWT, van der Vleuten CPM. Programmatic Assessment and Kane's Validity Perspective. *Medical Education*. 2012;46(1):38–48.

11. Tavares T, Brydges R, Myre P, et al. Applying Kane's Validity Framework to a Simulation Based Assessment of Clinical Competence. *Advances in Health Science Education Theory and Practice*. 2018;23(2):323–338.

12. Hatala R, Cook DA, Brydges R, Hawkins R. Constructing a Validity Argument for the Objective Structured Assessment of Technical Skills (OSATS): A Systematic Review of Validity Evidence. *Advances in Health Sciences Education: Theory and Practice*. 2015;20(5):1149–1175.

13. Royal College of General Practitioners. MRCGP Exam Overview. 2019. https://www.rcgp.org.uk/training-exams/mrcgp-exam-overview.aspx.

14. Lockyer J, Carraccio C, Chan M-K, et al. Core Principles of Assessment in Competency-Based Medical Education. *Medical Teacher*. 2017;39(6):609–616.

15. Norcini J, Anderson MB, Bollela V, et al. 2018 Consensus Framework for Good Assessment. *Medical Teacher*. 2018;40(11):1102–1109.

16. Hodges B, Paul R, Ginsburg S. Assessment of Professionalism: From Where Have We Come to Where Are We Going? An Update from the Ottawa Consensus Group on the Assessment of Professionalism. *Medical Teacher*. 2019;41(3):249–255.

17. Swanson DB, Clauser BE, Case SM. Clinical Skills Assessment with Standardized Patients in High-Stakes Tests: A Framework for Thinking about Score Precision, Equating, and Security. *Advances in Health Sciences Education*. 1999;4(1):67–106.

18. Turner JL, Dankoski ME. Objective Structured Clinical Exams: A Critical Review. *Family Medicine*. 2008;40(8):574–578.

19. Wood TJ, Pugh D. Are Rating Scales Really Better than Checklists for Measuring Increasing Levels of Expertise? *Medical Teacher*. 2020;42(1):46–51.

20. Homer M, Fuller R, Hallam J, Pell G. Shining a Spotlight on Scoring in the OSCE: Checklists and Item Weighting. *Medical Teacher*. 2020;42(9):1037–1042.

21. De Champlain AF, Pugh D, Regehr G. Standard Setting Methods in Medical Education: Taking the Sting Out of Assessment: Is There a Role for Progress Testing? *Understanding Medical Education*. 2016;50(7):347–359.

22. Yousuf N, Violato C, Zuberi RW. Standard Setting Methods for Pass/Fail Decisions on High-Stakes Objective Structured Clinical Examinations: A Validity Study. *Teaching and Learning in Medicine*. 2015;27(3):280–291.

23. Hejri SM, Jalili M, Muijtjens AMM, Van Der Vleuten CPM. Assessing the Reliability of the Borderline Regression Method as a Standard Setting Procedure for Objective Structured Clinical Examination. *Journal of Research in Medical Sciences*. 2013;18(10):887–891.

24. Homer M, Fuller R, Hallam J, Pell G. Setting Defensible Standards in Small Cohort OSCEs: Understanding Better When Borderline Regression Can "Work." *Medical Teacher*. 2020;42(3):306–315.

25. Homer M, Pell G, Fuller R, Patterson J. Quantifying Error in OSCE Standard Setting for Varying Cohort Sizes: A Resampling Approach to Measuring Assessment Quality. *Medical Teacher*. 2016;38(2):181–188.

26. Norcini JJ. Setting Standards on Educational Tests. *Medical Education*. 2003; 37(5):464–469.

27. Pell G, Fuller R, Homer M, et al. How to Measure the Quality of the OSCE: A Review of Metrics—AMEE Guide No. 49. *Medical Teacher*. 2010;32(10):802–811.

28. Fuller R, Homer M, Pell G. Longitudinal Interrelationships of OSCE Station Level Analyses, Quality Improvement and Overall Reliability. *Medical Teacher*. 2013;35(6):515–517.

29. Pell G, Fuller R, Homer M, et al. How to Measure the Quality of the OSCE: A Review of Metrics—AMEE Guide No. 49. *Medical Teacher*. 2010;32(10):802–811.

30. Fuller R, Homer M, Pell G, Hallam J. Managing Extremes of Assessor Judgment within the OSCE. *Medical Teacher*. 2017;39(1):58–66.

31. Pell G, Homer M, Fuller R. Investigating Disparity Between Global Grades and Checklist Scores in OSCEs. *Medical Teacher*. 2015;37(12):1106–1113.

32. Pell G, Fuller R, Homer M, Roberts T. Advancing the Objective Structured Clinical Examination: Sequential Testing in Theory and Practice. *Medical Education*. 2013;47(6):569–577.

33. Yeates P, Cope N, Hawarden A, et al. Developing a Video-Based Method to Compare and Adjust Examiner Effects in Fully Nested OSCEs. *Medical Education*. 2019;53(3):250–263.

34. Boursicot K, Kemp S, Wilkinson T, et al. Performance Assessment: Consensus Statement and Recommendations from the 2020 Ottawa Conference. *Medical Teacher*. 2020. doi:10.1080/0142159X.2020.1830052.

35. Ghouri A, Boachie C, McDowall S, et al. Gaining an Advantage by Sitting an OSCE After Your Peers: A Retrospective Study. *Medical Teacher*. 2018;40(11):1136–1142.

36. McKinley DW, Norcini JJ. How to Set Standards on Performance-Based Examinations—AMEE Guide No. 85. *Medical Teacher*. 2014;36(2):97–110.

37. Pugh D, Bhanji F, Cole G, et al. Do OSCE Progress Test Scores Predict Performance in a National High-Stakes Examination? *Medical Education*. 2016;50(3):351–358.

38. Pell G, Fuller R, Homer M, Roberts T. Is Short-Term Remediation After OSCE Failure Sustained? A Retrospective Analysis of the Longitudinal Attainment

of Underperforming Students in OSCE Assessments. *Medical Teacher*. 2012;34(2):146–150.

39. Conn CA, Bohan KJ, Pieper SL, Musumeci M. Validity Inquiry Process: Practical Guidance for Examining Performance Assessments and Building a Validity Argument. *Studies in Educational Evaluation*. 2020;65:100843.

40. Eweda G, Bukhary ZA, Hamed O. Quality Assurance of Test Blueprinting. *Journal of Professional Nursing*. 2020;36(3):166–170.

41. Hodges B. Validity and the OSCE. *Medical Teacher*. 2003;25(3):250–254.

42. St-Onge C, Young M. Evolving Conceptualisations of Validity: Impact on the Process and Outcome of Assessment. *Medical Education*. 2015;49(6):548–550.

43. Tannenbaum RJ, Kane MT. *Stakes in Testing: Not a Simple Dichotomy but a Profile of Consequences that Guides Needed Evidence of Measurement Quality*. ETS Research Report Series; 2019:1.

44. Karam VY, Park YS, Tekian A, Youssef N. Evaluating the Validity Evidence of an OSCE: Results from a New Medical School. *BMC Medical Education*. 2018;18(1):313.

45. General Medical Counseling. *Requirements for the Medical Licensing Assessment Clinical and Professional Skills Assessment*. 2019. https://www.gmc-uk.org/education/medical-licensing-assessment

46. ASPIRE. Areas of Excellence to Be Recognized. 2020. https://www.aspire-to-excellence.org/Areas+of+Excellence/

47. Hannon P, Lappe K, Griffin C, Roussel D, Colbert-Getz J. An Objective Structured Clinical Examination: From Examination Room to Zoom Breakout Room. *Medical Education*. 2020;54(9):864–861.

48. Lara S, Foster CW, Hawks M, Montgomery M. Remote Assessment of Clinical Skills During COVID19: A Virtual, High-Stakes, Summative Pediatric Objective Structured Clinical Examination. *Academic Paediatrics*. 2020;20(6):760–761.

49. Major S, Sawan L, Vognsen J, Jabre M. COVID-19 Pandemic Prompts The Development of a Web-OSCE Using Zoom Teleconferencing to Resume Medical Students' Clinical Skills Training at Weill Cornell Medicine–Qatar. *BMJ Simulation & Technology Enhanced Learning*. 2020.

50. Boursicot K, Kemp S, Ong TH, et al. Conducting a High-Stakes OSCE in a COVID-19 Environment. MedEdPublish. 2020.

51. Canning CA, Freeman KJ, Curran I, Boursicot K. Managing the COVID-19 Risk: The Practicalities of Delivering High Stakes OSCEs During a Pandemic. MedEdPublish. 2020.

52. Fuller F, Joynes V, Cooper J, Boursicot K, Roberts T. Could COVID-19 Be Our "There Is No Alternative" (TINA) Opportunity to Enhance Assessment? *Medical Teacher*. 2020;42(7):781–786.

5 Quality Assurance of Workplace Based Assessment

Karen E. Hauer, Jennifer R. Kogan, Patricia S. O'Sullivan, and Subha Ramani

CHAPTER HIGHLIGHTS

- This chapter defines workplace-based assessment (WBA) and characterizes its purpose within a program of assessment to describe learners' interactions with patients and teams and performance of essential tasks in the workplace.

- Many available tools for WBA exist, and educators select tools based on the skills deemed important to observe and feasibility and acceptability of the tool for the learners and observers in a particular educational and clinical context.

- Successful implementation of WBA requires a change in learning culture to promote learners' and supervisors' understanding of and skill with direct observation and feedback.

- Feedback represents dialogue centered within the learner–supervisor relationship where supervisors use WBA data to guide learners in reflecting on their performance, identifying gaps, and generating plans for improvement.

- Quality assurance of the WBA system requires communicating the purpose and use of WBA to participants, monitoring data quality, and creating and assessing a plan for aggregating data to make decisions about learner competence.

▌ ORIENTATION TO THE CHAPTER

This chapter focuses on the use of WBA as part of a program of assessment within a medical education curriculum. The chapter begins with a general overview and definitions of key terms related to WBA. The introduction is followed by a focus on feedback because effective feedback discussions are essential for learners to achieve learning benefit from WBA experiences. Training in effective feedback should emphasize the importance of placing the learner at the center of a feedback conversation and establishing trusting learner–teacher relationships for feedback to promote learner growth and performance change. Next, the chapter turns to implementation issues, including tool selection or development, and capturing information through ratings and narrative comments. Implementation considerations also tackle the many components of the context in which the tool is used, including the local culture, clinical and educational context, systems, people and technology. Introducing WBA into an educational program requires a robust communication plan so that educational program leaders, learners and teachers are aligned in their understanding of what is to be done, why it is being done, and how it should be done. Faculty and all assessors must receive training that includes expectations for learner performance, strategies to incorporate WBA into a clinical workflow, and methods of engaging in feedback discussions. The chapter concludes by addressing considerations for using WBA information to make judgments about learner performance and guide future learning, including how to synthesize information for these purposes. Programs must also attend to quality assurance by monitoring the data collected and procedures used. Case examples throughout the chapter serve as examples to illustrate key points about WBA.

INTRODUCTION

Defining Workplace-Based Assessment

Workplace-based assessment entails assessment of performance in practice [1]. WBA targets the highest level on Miller's pyramid of assessment [2]: What the learner does in actual practice (see Figure 4-1 from previous chapter). Collecting and collating information about trainees' or doctors' performance in their practice can occur through direct observation of actual work, such as a patient interaction, or observation of a work product, such as a patient note in a clinical record [3]. As snapshots of a learner's daily work, WBAs occur as single observations at a point in time. To provide meaningful representation of an individual's performance, broad sampling through repeated use of WBAs must occur to capture performance across contexts and over time to collectively contribute to valid judgments of performance.

Purpose of Workplace-Based Assessment

WBAs can serve several purposes. First, WBA can provide feedback to learners so that they understand how their current levels of performance compare to expected performances defined by outcome competencies.

During or after conducting a WBA, the assessor facilitates a feedback conversation combining learners' impressions of their own performance with their observation data. **Case 5-1** illustrates how WBA can ensure regular, ongoing feedback for students throughout their clerkships.

Second, the WBA serves to collect important data for a larger program of assessment [4]. A robust assessment system captures multiple data points with a range of assessment tools, including WBAs, to create a well-rounded view of the learner. Third, WBAs conducted for groups of learners within a training program can inform educational leaders about the effectiveness of the overall curriculum. For example, identification of strengths, areas for growth, or deficiencies within the aggregate WBA performance data can prompt curricular change to ensure that all learners are gaining the experiences needed to meet program expectations. Review of aggregate WBA data may also identify additional training needs for the WBA assessors to optimize their roles. Fourth, the direct observation, which occurs as part of WBA, can help inform how much supervision each learner requires to ensure that patients receive high-quality care.

WBA differs from other forms of assessment. Many traditional approaches to assessment occur outside the workplace, typically in settings designed specifically for assessment rather than patient care. Assessment of learner performance in decontextualized settings, such as occurs with written examinations of medical knowledge or simulated clinical encounters, allows for reproducible conditions to standardize the assessment. However, these assessments fail to incorporate the complexity and dynamic circumstances of the actual clinical environment. This complexity represents an essential feature of physician practice in which physicians and other providers must navigate different people, task variability, and competing demands each time they are in practice. WBAs also differ from global impressions of the learner obtained with an in-training evaluation form completed by a supervisor after a period of working together (i.e., end-of-rotation evaluation). In-training evaluations can capture useful information about performance but are limited compared to WBAs by recall bias and lack of specificity about particular interactions or tasks. Thus, multiple forms of assessments contribute unique and complementary information that, when combined, assures learners, educators, and the public about learners' achievement of competence for practice.

▌ CULTURE CHANGE

Promoting a Learning Culture to Facilitate WBA

Impactful use of WBA and the associated feedback dialogue require a culture supportive of this form of assessment. WBAs benefit from the

Case 5-1: WBA to Enhance Feedback for Students During Clerkships

Problem:

A medical student is surprised by her clerkship summary evaluation and grade. Her supervisors rarely observed her interacting with
patients or doing clinical tasks during her clerkship. Thus, she feels that
her supervisors' judgments were based only on their impressions of
her oral presentations on rounds. The feedback she received during
the clerkship was positive although quite general, without suggestions of actionable changes.

Solution:

Building on the principle of assessment for learning, the needed assessment to enhance the amount and usefulness of feedback would prompt
supervisors to observe the student conducting clinical work (e.g., history taking, physical exam, patient education, and counselling). In addition, a WBA tool to address these needs would engage supervisors and
students in formative discussions at the time of clinical work to provide
students with ongoing feedback so that they can make adjustments
and be observed again. Addressing the need for additional WBA begins
with clarifying expectations for learners and supervisors concerning
the nature and frequency of assessments and orienting to available
resources. The program adopts a WBA tool for observation of student's
patient care and communication skills and develops an app for recording feedback on a smartphone in real time. Program leaders create training materials (written instructions, video) describing use of the tool and
provide a video example of a student with a patient to be used by faculty to practice assessment and role play feedback discussions.

Take Home Message:

Students and faculty needed orientations and reminders to engage in
short observations and feedback discussions during patient care. The
WBA tool initially required completion on a desktop computer, a process
that led to delays in completing the form. The design of the smartphone
app, which entailed iterative discussion with potential users, leads
to a tool that is readily available and easy to use during clinical shifts.
Although faculty initially report difficulty incorporating observation
and feedback into clinical schedules, educating faculty and students on
WBAs and the process helps them collaborate to find opportune times.
Student satisfaction with feedback during clerkships improves.

organizational perspective of culture, characterized by Watling as "shared assumptions, beliefs and values that characterize a setting." Organizational culture has been described as the *social glue* that binds an organization or as the "collective programming of the mind" that distinguishes its members [5]. For WBAs to be successful, the culture must include shared assumptions about the importance of and communal responsibility for engaging in direct observation of learners and providing skilled feedback. For organizations or institutions where these elements are lacking, the organizational change literature provides key insights to facilitate culture change. For example, Kotter [6] argues for a process that includes incorporating a sense of urgency as to why WBAs are needed and the importance of a clear vision that is communicated widely. Also critical is leadership commitment to WBA implementation communicated through ongoing messaging about the central role of WBA and feedback in education while acknowledging the need to fit this activity into busy clinicians' workdays. Socializing the use of direct observation, the tool for WBA, and feedback entails repeated communications coupled with systems design that enable learners and clinicians to accomplish these tasks within the context of their other responsibilities. These strategies can together build a culture supportive of WBA.

Communicating the Purpose of WBA

Leadership must communicate the purpose of WBA, providing learners and their supervisors with a shared understanding of the intent and use of information derived from a WBA. A formative purpose is designed to inform the learner of progress compared to expectations, promote learner reflection, and guide learning plans [7]. Formative assessment can motivate learners by showcasing where and how they can improve their performance; assessment should be followed by the opportunity to reattempt a task. To see the value in WBA, learners require developmental feedback that highlights needed changes to performance and addresses how to fulfill these learning needs. In contrast, summative assessment entails using information collected as part of WBA or other assessment data to make judgments about a learner's competence and readiness for advancement.

Dual use of WBA to serve both formative and summative purposes simultaneously, no matter how well intended, typically fails to achieve these dual functions [8,9]. Learners tend to view assessments as summative regardless of the intent. When they perceive that a WBA has a summative purpose, learners alter their behavior and become strategic in showcasing their best performance [10]. This performance orientation may reflect learners' prior education in which high grades and scores were necessary to qualify for entry into medical school or residency. As such, aiming to use a WBA for both formative and summative purposes may be particularly unsuccessful in achieving the formative aim because learners will prioritize putting forth their strengths and hiding their limitations or learning needs.

Inclusion of WBA tools within a program of assessment codifies procedures for direct observation of learners and their work. Educators should design strategies to build direct observation into the clinical workflow to ensure its completion. However, direct observation of learners' performance in medical training historically has been infrequent. Learners and educators may avoid this activity for multiple reasons. Learners at multiple levels fear a resultant summative judgment; in undergraduate medical education, students commonly fear jeopardizing their grade if an assessor were to observe them performing less than optimally; and in postgraduate medical education, learners want to enjoy autonomy rather than direct supervision [11]. Faculty reticence to conduct direct observation may stem from insecurity about their own clinical skills and ability to teach those skills, time pressures generated by competing responsibilities, or the inability to assess learners effectively in the context of a brief observation [12]. Further, when direct observation of learner performance does occur, observations tend to be selective and focused on certain tasks or competencies while neglecting others [13]. **Case 5-1** illustrates how WBA can address these issues. Overall, thoughtful use of WBA within an educational program helps create a culture that maximizes the value of clinical learning, views direct observation and feedback as the norm, and encourages continuous improvement.

Tools for WBA

A variety of tools are available for WBA (Table 5-1). The individual conducting the assessment, referred to here as the *assessor*, can be one of many individuals in the workplace, including a supervisor, peer, interprofessional colleague, or even a patient. Competency-based medical education (CBME), in which the medical education program is designed to ensure learners' achievement of desired outcomes, requires defining the learning experiences and instruction necessary to progress toward those outcomes. WBA tools enable observation and focused feedback targeting expectations and activities in which learners participate.

Table 5-1 R2C2 FEEDBACK MODEL [17]	
Step 1— Relationships	• Prioritizes establishment of learner–teacher rapport and relationships as precursors to meaningful feedback conversations. • Rapport can be established regardless of the duration of an educational or working relationship through eliciting learner goals and establishing the context and purpose of the performance observation and ensuing feedback discussion.
Step 2— Reaction	• Focuses on eliciting learner reaction to the clinical encounter, both positive and negative, through open-ended questions.
Step 3— Content	• Content or observed events during the clinical encounter are discussed. • Ensures clarification about why learners carried out certain strategies or behaviors, ensures learner agreement with teacher observations that target change in learner behavior and practice. • Ends with the learner decision on one or two areas for improvement or change.
Step 4— Coaching for Growth	• Teacher helps the learner to formulate an action plan for improvement in areas that have been decided upon in step 3. • Teachers and learners discuss what the specific gaps in observed and expected performance might be and what strategies could narrow the gap.

▌ FEEDBACK

Feedback Principles: The Underpinnings of the What and Why

At the center of successful implementation of WBA is effective feedback to learners. Given that many of the precepts of effective feedback are foundational to WBA, this next section provides important background and application of feedback principles to practice for a program that includes WBA. Learner engagement in feedback conversations and trusting teacher–learner relationships increase the likelihood that learners will accept and incorporate feedback into their practice.

Feedback Definition

The dominant view in medical education is that feedback is a unidirectional flow of information from supervisor to learners for their future

Feedback data anchored in performance observation

Tone of feedback provider

Trusting relationships

Learner Self-efficacy/Positive face

Growth mindset

Limited teacher-learner relationships

Feedback provider and data perceived as lacking credibility

Fixed mindset

Desire for autonomy/Negative face

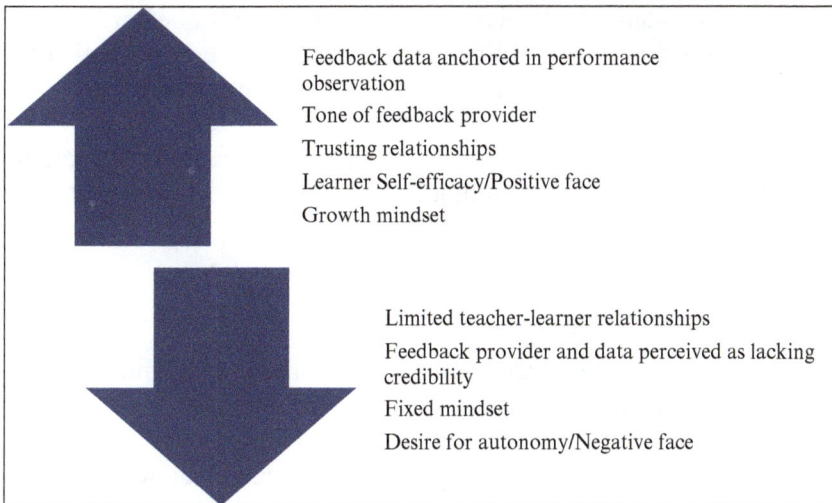

Figure 5-1 • Sociocultural factors that influence feedback acceptance.

performance improvement. Older definitions of feedback emphasize supervisors' skills in providing feedback—"information describing students' or residents' performance in a given activity that is intended to guide their future performance in the same activity" [14]. This understanding fails to incorporate the learner perspective or address the critical question of whether feedback is understood and accepted.

In the context of WBA, medical students and residents have reported infrequent and suboptimal quality of faculty feedback with little impact on subsequent performance. Clinical teachers also report several barriers to providing learners with feedback, including time constraints, inadequate skills in providing feedback, and fear of damaging teacher–learner relationships [13]. Learners and supervisors also may not view feedback through the same lens. Newer definitions and conceptualizations of feedback in medical education can facilitate a shared mental model of its purpose and process.

Newer Conceptualizations and Credibility Concepts

Newer definitions of feedback emphasize that feedback is only effective when the recipient accepts the information and makes a consequent behavior or practice change [14]. Recent research has generated a body of literature on rejection and acceptance of feedback by learners—that is, perceived credibility of the information by recipients [15,16]. Factors that influence credibility include the learners' relationships with feedback providers, the manner in which feedback is provided, whether the feedback was based on direct observation of performance, and whether the feedback content aligns with learners' impressions of their own performance. Thus, research has shifted focus toward feedback provider–recipient relationships and factors that promote feedback acceptance and change in behavior, including a focus on psychological safety and mindset [17].

Role of Feedback in CBME

Predicated on defining outcomes of training and then aligning training experiences to achieve those outcomes, competency-based medical education requires regular exchange of formative performance-based feedback during supervisor–learner discussion. This information allows learners to participate in self-assessment and formulate action plans to narrow any gaps between their current and expected performance. A safe feedback culture normalizes reflection on strengths and deficiencies as essential for learners to engage actively in this bidirectional process.

Goal Orientation and Mindset

In a culture that embraces feedback, supervisors establish a safe environment to encourage a growth mindset, elicit learning goals from learners, observe performance addressing those learning goals, and facilitate self-reflection. Teachers and learners alike need to view "failure" as a learning opportunity and not as an insult to self-esteem [18]. Feedback acceptance by learners is influenced by their own feedback-seeking behaviors, ability to accurately self-assess, goal orientation, and perceptions of threat to self-esteem [19]. Individuals with a performance goal orientation seek feedback to showcase excellence and tend to reject feedback perceived as negative or threatening to their self-esteem [8]. Institutions and supervisors can promote a learning goal orientation by emphasizing mastery of new knowledge and skills rather than appearance of excellence, an approach that aligns with the purpose of WBAs.

Sociocultural Principles and Feedback

Because feedback (and WBA) is increasingly viewed as a complex interpersonal encounter anchored in trusting working relationships, it is useful to view feedback through a sociocultural perspective. Sociocultural theory proposes that humans learn largely through social interactions influenced by cultural beliefs and attitudes [20]. Clinical learning occurs through team interactions and collaboration. Therefore, institutions should attend not only to the development of individual learners but also to the broader community in which learning is occurring. Applying these principles to feedback, educators need to (1) identify learner abilities using a developmental approach, (2) identify gaps between learners' current versus expected performance, and (3) engage team members and potentially patients to provide formative feedback.

Brown and Levinson's politeness theory proposes that two types of *face*—positive (one's need to be appreciated by others) and negative (one's desire for freedom of action)—play a role in most social interactions [21]. To save face, learners and supervisors may perceive constructive feedback as a breach of the norms of expected politeness, leading to avoidance of any discussion of gaps in performance. Thus, supervisors need to develop strategies for feedback conversations that can attend to self-esteem and also include honest constructive feedback [19]. Sociocultural factors that influence feedback acceptance are shown in Figure 5-1.

Two Learner-Centered Models for Framing Feedback Conversations

Most clinical supervisors are familiar with the importance of forming a therapeutic alliance with patients. The educational alliance is this concept applied to feedback [15]. A conducive educational alliance between teachers and learners can improve feedback acceptance and learner behavior change, the most important goals of feedback in WBA. Therefore, orienting teachers and learners to the importance of and strategies to establish an educational alliance is necessary before direct observation of and feedback on performance. Teachers and learners should co-construct such an alliance for maximal learner growth. Key strategies include establishment of a safe environment where strengths and weaknesses are normalized, expectations that conversations will include reinforcing and constructive feedback, discussion of learner goals with the teacher or assessor, observation of performance, and feedback conversations that stimulate the learner to reflect, self-assess, select a few areas for improvement, and create action plans and discrete next steps. Sargeant et al. proposed a model for feedback conversations titled relationships, reaction, content, and coaching (R2C2) [17], which similarly emphasizes learner engagement throughout a feedback conversation (Table 5-1). This model is anchored by teacher–learner relationships and the application of coaching principles.

> **Box 5-1   FEEDBACK STRATEGIES THAT ADDRESS SELF-ESTEEM AND AUTONOMY THROUGH MINIMIZATION OF THREATS TO "FACE"**
>
> Make direct observation a regular occurrence in the clinical workplace
>
> Train clinical teachers to observe their learners' performance without impeding their relationship with patients
>
> Establish goals for the observation and reach shared understanding on the purpose of these encounters and the feedback exchange
>
> Use language that is honest, based on behaviors with examples from the encounter, and facilitates self-reflection
>
> Allow learners to formulate action plans for improvement

Balancing Honest Feedback with Attention to Learner Self-Esteem and Autonomy

As previously mentioned, learners could perceive constructive feedback as a threat to self-esteem and direct observation as a threat to their autonomy. However, constructive feedback is more likely to result in performance improvement than nonspecific positive feedback [19]. Strategies to defuse threats to self-esteem and autonomy are illustrated in **Case 5-2** and Box 5-1.

Case 5-2 illustrates challenges related to the impact of feedback and the need for a shared mental model of feedback between teachers and learners.

> ### Case 5-2: WBA to Enhance Resident Feedback and Attend to "Face" in Continuity Clinic
>
> #### Problem:
>
> Many residents within an internal medicine residency program complain that the quality of feedback provided by their supervisors is poor and not based on credible performance data. The program pilots a direct observation initiative in the residents' continuity clinics by requesting that the longitudinal preceptors observe short segments of their resident–patient interactions at least three times a year. This leads to the paradox of enhancing the perceived credibility and quality of feedback but creating worry among residents and supervisors that this initiative might be impacting residents' autonomy and image projected to patients.
>
> #### Solution:
>
> Direct observation of performance is introduced to provide supervisors and residents with accurate data about their clinical performance.

Individual supervisors provide clear examples of performance to anchor feedback conversations, raising the feedback credibility. Training program leaders make periodic direct observations the norm, and this change prompts supervisors and residents to engage regularly in formative feedback conversations. Clinical supervisors and residents form an educational alliance and co-create action plans for performance improvement within coaching conversations structured around areas for improvement with one or two action plans and a strategy for follow-up. These changes shift the culture toward residents' greater comfort with feedback as helpful information rather than a threat to their autonomy. Patients come to view residents and supervisors as a team.

To make this change, the clinic adopts a WBA tool called *mini-CEX* for regular observation of resident–patient interactions by supervisors. Clinical leaders create training materials (handouts, videos, skills practice) for supervisors to provide training in direct observation, including observation behaviors that support learner autonomy, facilitation of self-assessment and reflection by residents, the co-creation of action plans, and coaching. For residents, training materials address feedback seeking and receiving and creating action plans for improvement. For both supervisors and residents, training addresses the importance of performance observation and feedback and establishing the climate to do this safely. Training for patients and families includes explaining the importance of direct observation for education.

Take Home Message:

Resident satisfaction with feedback improves, and educators observe improved resident skills in seeking feedback, reflecting on their own performance, and formulating action plans for improvement. Supervisors incorporate direct observation into the work routine, demonstrate attention to face, and enhance their coaching skills. Improved resident–supervisor working relationships raise the perceived credibility of feedback. Increased direct observation supports better supervision decisions, including supporting learner autonomy, and WBA is incorporated into the culture of the clinic.

Feedback language and content should align with ratings and assessment narratives. In conclusion, the practice of feedback in WBA should focus on helping the learner reflect, assess gaps between personal performance and expected performance in multiple clinical domains, and formulate plans for improvement as represented in Figure 5-2.

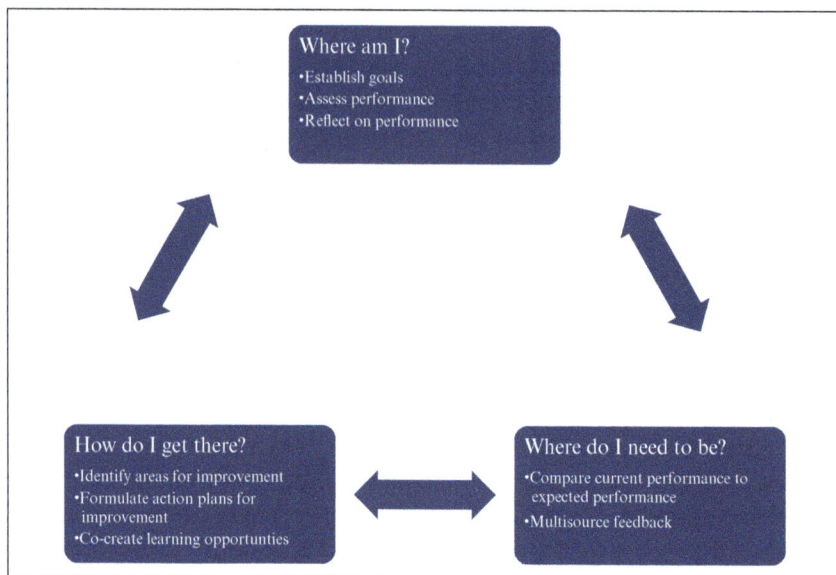

Figure 5-2 • Learner use of feedback to assess current versus expected performance

▌ WBA IMPLEMENTATION

Concepts related to culture and feedback set the stage for how to implement WBA. As previously discussed, WBA tools are used to anchor a feedback conversation based on observation of a learner's work by a supervisor. This section describes how to make decisions about tool selection and format, assessment platforms, and practical implementation considerations such as defining responsibility for WBA completion, promoting educational impact, and aligning work structures.

Broad Considerations and Requirements

Educators have many assessment tools available to assess learners in the clinical setting, particularly tools focused on history taking, physical exam, counseling, and procedural competence [22,23] (see Table 5-2). These tools can guide assessors' observations of the learner by scaffolding what behaviors and skills assessors should attend to. Tools also provide a mechanism to document observations. Given the availability of multiple tools, program leadership will need to decide which tool or tools to use. First and foremost are to determine whether the assessment tool is aligned with how the program intends to use it for learner feedback and assessment and how the instrument fits into the overall program of assessment of learner competence.

Table 5-2   COMMON TOOLS USED FOR DIRECT OBSERVATION OF CLINICAL SKILLS [22,23]

Tool Name	Skills or Competencies Assessed
Nonprocedural Tools	
Calgary–Cambridge	History taking, communication
Direct Observation Clinical Encounter Examination (DOCEE)	History taking, physical exam, communication, overall
Direct Observation of Clinical Skills (DOCS)	History taking, physical exam, oral case presentation
Minicard	History taking, professional conduct, physical exam, data synthesis or reasoning, interpersonal and communication skills, medical knowledge, professionalism, systems-based practice
Mini-Clinical Evaluation Exercise (mini-CEX)	History taking, physical exam, counselling, clinical reasoning, organization and efficiency, professionalism, overall impression
Professionalism mini-evaluation exercise	Doctor–patient relationship, reflective skills, time management, interpersonal communication skills
SEGUE	History taking, counselling
Structured clinical observation (SCO)	History taking, physical exam, counselling
Procedural Tools	
Direct observation of procedural skills (DOPS)	Critical knowledge, consent, preparation, vigilance, infection control, technical ability, patient interaction, insight, documentation, postprocedure management, team interaction
Global rating scale (GRS)	Respect for tissue, time and motion, knowledge of procedure, flow of procedure, and forward planning
Nontechnical skills for surgeons (NOTSS)	Situation awareness, decision-making, communication and teamwork, leadership
Objective structured assessment of technical skills (OSATS)	Respect for tissue, time and motion, instrument handling, knowledge of instruments, use of assistants, flow of operation, knowledge of specific procedure
Procedure-based assessment (PBS)	Consent, preoperative planning, preoperative preparation, exposure and closure, intraoperative technique, postoperative management

The effectiveness of WBA is realized when learners are observed while engaged in authentic work. Educational program leadership should identify the skills to be observed to inform competency assessments. Clinicians can provide input based on their firsthand experience with real-life skills required for delivering quality care. Learners have an important role in determining the focus of direct observation so that observation aligns with the specific skills they wish to develop.

WBA requires multiple observations to capture the scope of a learner's performance. Competence is not generic; it is specific to particular contexts and situations [24]. As such, WBAs must be sampled widely by observing learners in multiple different contexts and at multiple points in time, and by multiple different assessors. In a study of resident assessment using three WBA tools, sufficient reliability (coefficient of 0.80) was obtained with eight mini-CEXs and nine direct observation of procedural skills (DOPS) forms [25]. Taken together, these observations constitute information sufficient to create a rich and robust "picture" of the learner [24,26]. The WBA assessment tool may address competencies such as data gathering, procedures, and patient communication. **Case 5-3** illustrates how a WBA tool improves procedural skills learning by guiding learners and supervisors through planning, enactment, and discussion of direct observation in the surgical context.

The use of WBA requires an understanding of how the collection of performance information yields this rich picture. Direct observation tools are not simple checklists that record what a learner does or does not do. Assessment in the workplace is challenged by low reliability, meaning that the learner may perform differently, better or worse, on WBAs in different contexts, at different points in time or with different assessors. Nevertheless, the assessment has validity because it is situated in the workplace that has real, albeit variable, contexts. Variable contexts occur because of complex relationships between learners and their patients, learners and their assessors, and the nature of each clinical case and setting, which can vary day to day, clinical unit to clinical unit, and clinical site to clinical site. Therefore, the goal of WBA is not simply to measure learning outcomes but to understand how and what learners have learned and done [27]. Lastly, decisions about the amount of information that needs to be gathered by WBAs are tied to the stakes of the decision being rendered. When there are no or low stakes in the assessment, one data point focused on information to provide feedback is sufficient. However, to identify a learner's trajectory requires a number of WBAs. When stakes are high, such as in promotion or selection decisions, multiple data points are needed.

Case 5-3: WBA to Enhance Procedural Skills Feedback for Residents

Problem:

A resident is reviewed at the clinical competency committee. She has completed all required assessments in the surgical skills center. However, in the end-of-rotation evaluations, one division notes that she was not gentle with the tissue. When the program director meets with the resident, the resident is unclear as to what is meant by being "ungentle" and when and how this observation occurred.

Solution:

The resident needs timely feedback in authentic situations to help improve performance (assessment for learning). To address this need, program directors set clear expectations that attending surgeons will complete an operative skills assessment and review the assessment with the resident. The resident is then expected to devise strategies to work on the identified gap. During a rotation, advisors in the rotation help the resident examine the trajectory of performance using data review. Faculty provide feedback to skills lab educators about technical skills requiring more extensive training for this resident and potentially others.

Surgical educators use forms available from the American College of Surgeons with modifications as needed. They develop (or purchase) apps to allow assessment data acquisition. To communicate the new educational strategy, they host brief training sessions by video and in grand rounds.

In the operating room (OR), a preop discussion during the "time out" focuses each assessment. In a postop brief, the attending surgeon and resident review the surgery and the key skills in the portion of the surgery in which the resident was active. Making time for these discussions requires a scheduling strategy and cooperation from OR or operating theatre staff.

Take Home Message:

The attending surgeon and resident agree on the target for feedback. The resident receives input aimed at improving skills. An advisor helps the resident synthesize the overall performance because the operative experiences are not longitudinal with any one surgeon. This advisor invites the learner to engage in critical reflection. The OR staff engage in the process by allowing time for goal setting and feedback. Initial compliance with the new expectation is low. Subsequently, department leaders initiate communications about the importance of WBA, and a program administrator monitors WBA completion and sends reminders to residents and faculty. These efforts increase WBA completion.

WBA Tool Selection

Utility Index

Given the availability of multiple WBA tools, program directors may want guidance on selecting the most appropriate ones. The *utility index* is a useful framework that considers validity, reliability, acceptability, educational impact, and cost-effectiveness [28,29]. Each factor depends on the context in which the tool is used. Validity evidence demonstrates that the tool is measuring the intended construct of clinical skill and competence. Acceptability and cost-effectiveness influence feasibility. Educational impact is based in part on the educational and catalytic effects of the assessment. Norcini describes educational effect as whether and how the "assessment motivates those who take it to prepare in a fashion that has educational benefit" [29]. Catalytic effect is the way that "the assessment provides results and feedback in a fashion that creates, enhances, and supports education and drives future learning forward" [29]. Several systematic reviews summarize utility index factors for different WBA instruments [23,30,31]. This utility information should be considered in the context of the larger assessment system. WBAs may be best viewed as components of a system of assessment with strengths in validity and educational impact that approaches reliability through presenting information from broad sampling, multiple methods, multiple assessors, and multiple events over time to a panel of judges [32].

Intrarater and inter-rater reliability are a challenge with WBA tools. This variability is explained predominantly by variance among assessors [33], who bring differing clinical, educational, and assessment competence. In addition, exploration of rater cognition reveals that assessors demonstrate idiosyncrasy, make variable inferences, and are constrained by working memory and processing limitations, cognitive load, and subconscious processes such as bias and stereotyping [34]. A common yet erroneous response to these concerns is to create a new or change an existing tool or form to achieve greater intra- and inter-rater reliability. However, in WBA, the true assessment instrument is the assessor, not the tool. Therefore, assessor training is essential because assessment tools are only as good as the individual using them. Observer judgment underpins good assessment. Programs should avoid or minimize time and effort on new tool development; rather, they should direct resources toward selecting an existing tool and conducting assessor training. Maximizing the accuracy and quality of observation and feedback necessitates faculty development and rater training, which are discussed later in this chapter.

WBA Tool Formats

WBA tools differ in the skills they assess and how assessments are made. Tool features vary in the use of global ratings versus checklists, the rating scale or anchors used, the capture of quantitative versus qualitative data, and platform (written versus electronic). The choice of instrument depends primarily on the objectives of the teaching or assessment exercise.

Global Ratings versus Checklists: Some assessment tools such as the mini-CEX ask assessors to select global ratings (i.e., a rating for history taking, physical exam, or overall clinical skills). Other tools use checklists in which the assessor indicates whether specific behaviors were performed (e.g., items for history taking may include agenda setting, asking open-ended questions, responding to patient's nonverbal cues, etc.). Examples of tools using checklists include the SEGUE and the Calgary–Cambridge model [35,36]. Checklists may help assessors identify whether learners have performed, omitted, or performed incorrectly specific activities. This information can facilitate targeted feedback to learners. However, creating highly detailed checklists for every type of patient encounter is not feasible. Longer checklists may increase cognitive load and impede the number of relevant behaviors that assessors are able to identify. Consequently, they lose the capacity to differentiate between performance levels. The unintended consequence may lower inter-rater reliability.

Rating Scales and Anchors: WBA tools use different rating scales. Some scales contain numerical ratings with associated anchors. Anchors might be *unsatisfactory*, *satisfactory*, or *superior*. Other instruments have normative anchors such as *below expectation*, *at expectation*, and *exceeds expectation*. Some forms have behavioral anchors with behavioral descriptions of a skill associated with each number on the rating scale. Rating scale anchors based on supervision and entrustment are increasingly in use. These rating scales are either coparticipatory or supervisory, as shown in Table 5-3. These entrustment scales have several potential benefits. First, they may align cognitively with how supervisors think about their supervisory role and thus resonate with their experience. When prompted to consider their own supervision and entrustment, assessors are likely to discriminate between learners and thus avoid leniency. Second, these scales can therefore help increase the identification of learners performing below expectations. Third, there may be less interrater variability using these types of scales that, in turn, can decrease the number of assessments required to ensure reliable assessment. Unfortunately, current research has generated little evidence to determine the best scale anchors to use on these assessment tools. However, paramount above and beyond the tool chosen is the training and development of assessors to decrease variance in ratings [33].

Quantitative Versus Qualitative Data: Many direct-observation tools prompt assessors to provide narrative comments. When well written and based on directly observed behaviors or work products, narrative comments can provide learners with useful information about what they are doing well and how they can improve. Narrative comments make quantitative or checklist ratings actionable and can provide unique content to guide performance improvement. In general, when WBA is used for feedback, rich narrative comments that focus on behaviors are essential.

Assessment Platform: WBAs can be implemented using a paper-based or electronic system for data capture. The availability of web-based or app-based WBA instruments is increasing; many educators have developed smartphone-based systems to evaluate learners after they interact with patients or perform procedures. Electronic systems often include the option to dictate feedback. Electronic platforms can provide assessors

Table 5-3 COPARTICIPATORY AND SUPERVISORY SCALES COMPARED			
Coparticipatory Scale (Ottawa):		**Supervisory Scale (ten Cate):**	
How much the supervisor had to contribute in order for the task to be completed		Assessor prediction about how much supervision the learner would need next time if asked to do a similar task	
Rating	Descriptor	Rating	Descriptor
1	"I had to do."	1	"Not allowed to practice the EPA."
2	"I had to talk them through."	2	"Allowed to practice EPA only under proactive, full supervision."
3	"I had to prompt them from time to time."	3	"Allowed to practice EPA only under reactive, on demand supervision."
4	"I needed to be in the room just in case."	4	"Allowed to practice EPA unsupervised."
5	"I did not need to be there."	5	"Allowed to supervise others in practice of the EPA."

Sources: Gofton W, Dudek N, Wood T, Balaa F, Hamstra S. The Ottawa surgical competency operating room evaluation (O-SCORE): A tool to assess surgical competence. *Acad Med.* 2012;87:1401–1407; ten Cate O, Hart D, Ankel F, et al. Entrustment Decision Making in Clinical Training. *Acad Med.* 2016;91:191–198.

access to aggregated data showing how much experience a learner has with a given skill in order to individualize learning and feedback.

There are pros and cons to electronically based platforms when compared to paper formats. Some early studies suggest such WBA systems are acceptable and increase the ability to provide detailed feedback. Electronic platforms can be efficient for collecting, storing, and aggregating assessments. However, caution regarding security concerns and the privacy of the learner and potentially patient data is needed, and any system should be carefully vetted with information technology experts at the institution. Regardless of format, the WBA must be coupled with the social interaction that is essential for a feedback conversation.

WBA Implementation Considerations

Effective WBA requires multiple assessments in multiple contexts by multiple assessors at multiple points in time. Therefore, education program directors need to decide what skills need to be observed and assessed by whom, in what context, and in what clinical rotations or placements. Program leadership should determine how they will monitor whether observation is happening and of whom and by whom. They also need to plan how assessments are collated and interpreted. Key implementation considerations for faculty and learners are shown in Table 5-4.

For implementation, electronic platforms permit facile data aggregation by learner and assessor. Electronic portfolios can summarize which skills learners have performed under what supervision levels and provide early detection of a learner's strengths and areas requiring improvement so that faculty can provide support as needed. Similarly, learners can use synthesized data to monitor and inform their learning. Synthesized information can be used by competence committees, grading committees, and other educators making decisions about learners' progress and readiness for advancement in the program or to graduation. In addition, aggregated information across learners can be used to inform program and curricular change.

Regardless of how assessments are collected, decisions and policies are needed about who "owns" the data (for example, individual assessors, learners, or curricular leaders). Similarly, decisions about with whom data can or cannot be shared and how often data can be accessed (ad hoc, quarterly, annually, etc.) are essential. Given the time and resource limitations facing most programs, leadership must contemplate whether WBA will add to or replace existing assessment activities.

Table 5-4 KEY TOPICS FOR FACULTY AND LEARNER TRAINING		
Concept	**Faculty**	**Learners**
Purpose	Purpose of the WBA for formative or summative assessment within a program of assessment	Purpose of the WBA for formative or summative assessment within a program of assessment
Shared mental model	What the skill looks like when done well	What the skill looks like when done well
Implementation	Who can initiate the WBA and how? What clinical activities should be observed? What technology may be used to record WBAs?	Who can initiate the WBA and how? How to request WBA targeted to one's learning needs? What technology may be used to record WBAs?
Rating scale	How to understand and apply the rating scale on the WBA tool	How to interpret ratings of performance using the rating scale on the WBA tool
Narrative comments	How to construct high-quality, behavior-based comments that address program competencies or objectives	How to interpret and use narrative comments about one's performance to guide personal learning and improvement
Feedback	Principles of conveying observations to a learner	How to solicit and incorporate feedback; how to manage the emotional response after receiving corrective feedback
Direct observation	How to behave in the room when doing direct observation	How to interact with patients while being directly observed by a supervisor

Determining Responsibility

Implementation requires decisions regarding who is responsible for initiating WBA: assessors, learners, or both. Assigning responsibility to assessors may signal the importance of direct observation in the program, but learners may perceive that assessment is happening *to* and not *for* them. Assigning responsibility to learners empowers them to advance their skill development proactively. However, assessors who fail to observe when requested quickly undermine a learner-driven approach. WBA is optimized when both assessors and learners take mutual responsibility and ownership of the process; that is, assessors initiate direct observation on important and relevant skills, and learners have the agency to request observation that provides feedback in skills self-assessed as important for individual professional development.

Promoting Educational Impact

The educational impact of WBA is influenced by the approach to implementation [37]. Lorwald et al. developed a model to demonstrate how mini-CEX and Direct Observation of Procedural Skills (DOPS) implementation influenced the learner. Their model includes factors related to work structure, instruments, organizational culture, and users, as shown in Table 5-5. Above all, organizational culture must value teaching, a growth mindset and mastery learning based on deliberate practice, feedback, and coaching [37]. Assessors and learners should understand the purpose of direct observation and feedback and their co-responsibility for ensuring that it occurs. The educational impact of WBA is optimized when learners

Table 5-5	FACTORS THAT FACILITATE AND HINDER IMPLEMENTATION OF WBA
Factor	**Components**
Organizational culture	• Value of teaching and feedback • Importance of direct observation
Work structure	• Time for teaching and feedback • Faculty development • Career paths for educators • Curricula for trainees • Trainees' rotations
Instruments	• Snapshots of trainee performance vs. longitudinal assessment • Content of assessment (assessment below competence level vs. assessment of appropriate and relevant tasks)
Users	• Responsibilities in learning and teaching • Knowledge about the use and purpose of the tools • Supervisors' interest in medical education relationship between trainees and supervisors

*Factors identified in a focus group study of mini-CEX and DOPS tools

reflect on performance during direct observation and then receive high-quality, specific, relevant, and actionable feedback.

Aligning Work Structures

Effective direct observation requires a work environment with supportive work structures that specify and protect time for observation and feedback and the development of career paths for interested and skilled assessors. Staffing models for teaching and patient care should be appropriately adjusted to enable time for both observation and feedback. Effective implementation maximizes assessment of learners over time so that growth can be assessed longitudinally and feedback credibility and trustworthiness can be maximized [38]. Longitudinal learner–teacher relationships situate the assessment in the context of the learner's development [39] but could prompt favorable ratings to preserve the relationship. Less familiar evaluators may seem to be more objective than longitudinal evaluators but could also have less familiarity with what to observe in the context of the learner's trajectory and could be more intimidating. Balancing these two types of observer relationships may capitalize on the strengths and limitations of each. This optimization of supervisor to learner interactions necessitates thoughtful consideration of clinical assignments and rotations.

▌ COMMUNICATION AND WBAs

The preceding sections stressed the need for communication. WBAs are successful only in the context of a shared vision among the various stakeholders, including assessors, learners, and patients. In this section, communication is highlighted along with specific communication messages for each stakeholder group and suggested communication strategies.

The Role of Communication

The educational impact of WBA requires development of assessors and learners. Among Kotter's admonitions regarding failed culture change is undercommunicating [6]. Although educators can justify the usefulness of WBA and identify the numerous approaches to such assessments, learners, faculty, staff, and patients may vary in their level of understanding and thus thwart successful implementation. Not all faculty recognize the importance of WBA or have the skills to do it effectively. Buy-in from learners is equally essential. Some learners readily accept and value WBA, but many find it anxiety provoking and do not perceive it to be meaningful for their professional growth. Leadership will therefore need to orient assessors and learners to WBA and continuously address barriers undermining uptake. Leadership will also need to identify and protect the time for this development activity to occur. In addition, assessor training, as will be discussed, helps ensure that mutually agreed-upon clear standards defining competence are used and quality narratives are generated. Leadership will need to ensure that assessors have protected time for upfront training and longitudinal practice.

Communication to Clinical Faculty

All faculty must receive the following key communication messages to enable meaningful use of WBAs: The organization places an importance on feedback; faculty will receive orientation to the local WBA including how learners and the organization will use information from the WBA; and faculty will receive training in providing quality feedback. The logistics are often a stumbling block for successful implementation. What is clear to leadership is often unclear to those who have to do WBAs. Tables 5-4 and 5-5 present key topics to address in a straightforward manner for successful local implementation. The preparation of clinical faculty to conduct assessments and provide feedback should be improving with the emphasis on teaching qualifications in higher education now implemented in much of Europe. However, there is limited research on whether this preparation relates to faculty performance of WBAs.

The orientation to the locally used WBA has four components. First, learners and assessors receive an introduction that includes the WBA purpose and how learners and educational leaders use the data. Second, participants review logistics of using the WBA, including any technology. A discussion of logistics should also include explaining to assessors the importance of explicitly establishing a relationship and discussing trust with learners. Third, assessors should receive skills training in direct observation and quality feedback. Skills training for direct observation is an essential component of orientation. Faculty worry about how intrusive they are in observing, where and how to position themselves to observe, and how long to observe. The literature provides guidance for direct observation issues and training [40]. Faculty will need to review the WBA form and be guided in how to complete it. As discussed later in this chapter, faculty should receive training in how to mitigate bias that might occur in a WBA. Faculty may also need instruction and skills training to give quality feedback, including addressing the learner's emotions [41]. While we have cast feedback as a dialogue requiring skill, feedback may also be written—and that requires specific training to be informative and without bias. Finally, orientation should include information about whether assessors will receive feedback about their performance of WBAs. Leadership should consider whether assessors will receive individual feedback or group data such as how many of what types of WBAs were completed. Individual assessors should receive feedback and coaching if their data are discrepant or inadequate for the purpose of the WBA.

Communication to Learners

Like faculty members who manifest the organization's commitment to WBA, learners need to receive clear messages about the purpose, data use, and logistics of WBAs. They need clarification about the role of the WBAs and how the data are to be used, what assessors expect from learners, and what learners expect from assessors. Communication should emphasize that learners must become feedback seekers to gain full value of the WBA. Communication with learners focuses on ensuring that they have skills for asking for, receiving, and discussing feedback, including how to manage their emotional response to feedback and developing plans to monitor and improve performance based on the feedback. This communication can tie to skills in self-directed learning and reflection. For example, learners may use the feedback from a WBA to develop a SMART goal that they can strive to meet before another WBA. Communication with learners should connect how the WBA links to the competencies they should be demonstrating. The skill of incorporating feedback to improve practice falls under the scholar role in the CanMEDs framework from the Canadian Royal College of Physicians and Surgeons and the domain of practice-based learning and improvement in the Accreditation Council of Graduate Medical Education competencies.

Communication to learners must also address their concerns. As previously discussed, most individuals do not like feeling that they are being judged and may question the credibility of the feedback. In orientation to WBAs, framing the importance of a feedback dialogue may promote learner comfort with the WBA. Communications should emphasize that learners who are able to make reasonable self-assessments are able to take advantage of the feedback in the WBA. Additional resources should be available for learners who feel that the WBA data does not align with their own perceptions. Taken together, these strategies promote learners' buy-in and effective use of WBAs for performance improvement.

Communication to Others

The need for robust communication is not limited to faculty and learners. Other potential assessors for WBAs—including interprofessional learners or providers, near peers, and staff—need information as to why their input is sought. This broad participant list suggests that a breadth of communication tactics is required to engage assessors in the WBA and feedback culture. They will have some of the same questions as anyone else: What is the purpose? What am I to do? What happens with the data? Will I receive training? The overall message should be that WBAs allow learners to receive feedback from a variety of relevant individuals while engaging in authentic activities.

Communications to Patients and Families

In clinical settings, an important stakeholder in the direct observation exercise is the patient or family member. Box 5-2 shows strategies to ensure patient safety and quality of care during WBA. At teaching hospitals and clinics, most patients and families are aware that a team comprising practicing physicians as well as trainees provides clinical care. When conducting a direct observation of performance, the assessor steps back from the direct line of vision of the patient and adopts a fly-on-the-wall approach. Patients and family members need to be oriented to the purpose of the exercise and why a senior clinician is observing and taking notes without participating in the clinical discussion. Yet the assessor must validate and give appropriate autonomy to the trainee as a care provider. When asked questions from patients or family members, assessors should gently redirect questions to trainees, thus cementing their roles as the primary clinician. If assessors are also part of a patient care team, they should note any agreement with the trainee's diagnostic plans as appropriate while offering alternative approaches where the trainee's plans may not be accurate. Finally, clinical supervisors should solicit feedback from patients whenever possible to demonstrate their respect, the patient centeredness of the exercise, and their commitment to shared decision-making.

Box 5-2   STRATEGIES TO ENSURE PATIENT SAFETY AND PATIENT CARE QUALITY DURING DIRECT OBSERVATION

- Orientation of patients and families to the team-based model of care
- Reassurance that a seasoned clinician is continuously monitoring diagnostic decision-making
- Showcasing direct observation as a quality assurance exercise
- Obtaining patient feedback on performance
- Concluding every encounter with explanations, clarification of jargon, and questions from patients
- Obtaining patient perspective and engaging in shared decision-making

Communication Strategies

Multiple communication strategies can reinforce key messages. Signage reminds everyone in the clinical setting about the feedback culture and completion of WBAs. Short videos or podcasts can elaborate implementation details. Additional communication about the assessor's role in WBAs are tailored to the assessor group. For example, patients complete a WBA to enhance quality of care in the future. Staff can be encouraged to complete WBAs to help a learner and to provide information to the program that may lead to a redesign of workplace experiences. Near peers have cognitive congruence with the learner and may provide insightful feedback tailored to the learner's development. Each assessor should be assured that the data is either confidential or anonymous. Communication about how these occasional assessors contributes to learners' development, and needed program changes provide assurance of the value of WBAs.

▌AVOIDING COMMON PITFALLS

WBA may seem to be a straightforward addition to a program of assessment, but successful implementation requires careful planning and ongoing monitoring. Educators may succumb to the pitfall of searching for the right tool as a guarantee of successful adoption of WBA. However, the tool must be selected for a particular purpose in the local context; lack of alignment between the tool and the purpose will undermine the impact of assessment. In addition to tool selection, educators must attend to faculty and learner preparation for using the tool. Commonly, insufficient attention is given to the feedback skills that will be needed for both faculty and learners to engage in meaningful feedback discussions within trusting relationships that can produce change in future learner behavior. Another pitfall in WBA implementation addresses data collection and data management. The use of WBA tools can generate plentiful quantitative and qualitative data that can be cumbersome for learners and education program leaders to synthesize and interpret. To avoid this pitfall, educators should identify a platform for storing and synthesizing electronic performance data and support learners with knowledgeable coaches or advisors who can help them use the information to make learning plans for improvement. A quality assurance pitfall arises when there is failure to monitor the completion and quality of WBAs and intervention is subsequently required to address gaps or deficiencies so as to optimize WBA.

▮ MONITORING AND EVALUATION

Having described WBA, implementation considerations, communication messages, and strategies, including around newer conceptualizations of feedback, as well as pitfalls, this last section of the chapter addresses quality assurance through monitoring and evaluation of the program. Quality assurance monitors the processes used and achievement of desired outcomes. This section focuses on communication about a quality assurance system for WBA; how to aggregate WBA; how to use them as data presented to competency, grading, or advancement committees; and how to monitor for assessment quality. Gaps in process and outcomes provide targets for improvement efforts.

Communication: Systems Change and Quality Assurance of the WBA Program

For quality assurance to be successful, learners and faculty should be informed of the system to monitor WBAs to ensure that WBAs are meeting the educational goals expected. Quality assurance needs to determine if communication, as previously described, is occurring to the extent planned because that communication forms the core of creating the desired WBA culture—willingness to observe and to give feedback, and willingness to be observed and receive feedback. One approach to quality assurance is to incorporate the notion of "feedback detailing" so that roles and responsibilities for feedback can be normalized into the culture [42]. The business literature showcases how a feedback culture is critical to improving individual job performance. In an organization with a strong feedback culture, feedback is valued, individuals are trained to give feedback, and individuals are supported to use feedback to improve [43]. Quality assurance must monitor that this culture is being created and that systems are in place to ensure that learners, clinical faculty and staff, interprofessional providers, peers and near peers, and patients are aware of the culture.

The quality assurance system should prompt questions related to the WBA process: Are individuals oriented? Are WBAs completed at the planned level? Are all types of assessors participating? Are learners engaged in the process? The quality assurance system must monitor that the time and place for orientation and the associated training are available. The quality assurance system must determine if the WBAs are occurring and with the quality planned and that learners are using the data. Analysis of data collected can determine the frequency and timing of WBAs. Quality assurance can be done by sampling feedback comments and assessing them using rubrics for feedback quality. Also, learner SMART goals can be reviewed to assess alignment with feedback comments to determine how well feedback is driving learning planning. Although complex, these monitoring tasks are feasible. However, they may require policies to ensure that WBAs are used for the intended purpose in the intended way. At the program level, the quality assurance system should address whether data aggregation is sufficiently informative for decision-making groups and the ways in which groups make those decisions.

Data Aggregation

WBA entails collecting large amounts of data across a range of assessors and contexts. Together, this information becomes part of a program of assessment, a centrally coordinated approach to assessment [44]. Whereas each WBA encounter constitutes only one data point, each provides important feedback to the learner. The aggregate collection of WBA information, combined with other assessment data from written examinations, clinical simulations, in training evaluations, or other tools, provides a rich description of each learner's performance across contexts and over time [4]. A mechanism is needed to synthesize this large amount of information. The purpose of synthesis is to demonstrate to the learner and to the learner's faculty advisor, coach, teacher, or mentor that the the learner is progressing overall. Leadership can use this information to make judgments about readiness for advancement or unsupervised practice.

An electronic method of aggregating performance information facilitates continuous monitoring of performance by facilitating understanding of each learner's learning history and trajectory. For example, an electronic learner dashboard provides comprehensive high-level, data-driven summaries that serve as actionable performance information. A useful dashboard is more than a data warehouse. To help learners and faculty make sense of performance data, the dashboard becomes an information-management system to process and display synthesized information [45]. Such a platform also enables drill-down views for detailed information, both quantitative and qualitative, about particular data or events such as a WBA. Displayed information about performance may be compared relative to expected benchmarks (criteria) or relative to group performance of peers (normative). A portfolio is a collection of a learner's work [3]. Typically, a learner populates the portfolio with a variety of work products that all together show evidence of performance and progress. The portfolio prompts the learner to reflect on learning and progress and set goals for further learning and improvement.

From a quality assurance perspective, the benefits of *big data*—the large data set stemming from use of WBAs—are shown through elucidating use of WBA within an education program. Learning analytics, the collection and review of data about how learning activities and behaviors occur within an education program, can reveal how early and consistently learners collect WBAs [46,47]. Patterns of learner behavior may emerge for individuals or groups of learners that indicate intrinsic or extrinsic motivation to complete WBAs. For example, are learners collecting WBAs in time to make changes to their performance within a particular context? From the assessor perspective, learning analytics can similarly reveal which assessors engage with the program, the types of ratings they provide, whether they use the full rating scale available, the length or depth of their narrative comments, and the timing of their WBAs. These data can inform further faculty training and adjustments to the system so that WBAs are feasible for assessors alongside their clinical responsibilities.

Competence Committees

Competence committees are now a required component of performance review in Canada, where the Royal College of Physicians and Surgeons Competence by Design introduced a requirement for competence committees, as well as in the United States, where Accreditation Council for Graduate Medical Education [47] requirements mandate clinical competency committees in all graduate medical education training programs. Competence committees use information from WBAs and other assessment tools to review and synthesize performance information about individual learners to make determinations about each learner's progress. Similarly, grading committees synthesize performance information for students to determine grades [48].

The competence committee benefits from a range of information. The importance of ensuring a broad sampling of WBAs across contexts, cases, assessors cannot be underestimated. **Case 5-4** describes how a competence committee incorporates multisource feedback to enhance its understanding of residents' work and improve their learning in the ambulatory clinic setting. The committee can adjudicate an outlier low-performance rating or negative narrative comment by considering the information in the context of all of the available information for that learner.

A component of quality assurance addresses the degree to which the committee members feel that they have sufficient data to make an informed assessment of each learner's growth. Determination of sufficiency capitalizes on the number of WBAs and also the quality of the narrative comments and range of skills or competencies captured. The committee also relies on the sufficiency of its own methods of data aggregation, interpretation, and synthesis to judge learners' progress. The committee or decision-making body has a responsibility to bolster the system by providing feedback regarding the need to alter or enhance training systems to optimize data collection and guidance to learners.

Educators using aggregate WBA data will question whether the information enables them to discriminate learners and their performance. As part of programmatic assessment within a CBME program, educators and learners shift their focus away from normative comparison of learners to one another for purposes of ranking and sorting them. Rather, the comparison of learners is against expected criteria or standards of performance. Accordingly, with WBA, it is important that programs articulate the criteria for performance in the activities observed using WBA. Learners and their educators may use WBA to discriminate one learner's individual relative strengths and areas for improvement. In addition, how the learner uses the WBA data can inform how that learner pursues improvement and enacts lifelong learning skills, and thus discern residents who demonstrate those skills.

Over time, program leaders can assess whether WBA is enhancing learning. Educators must be able to determine whether learners who aren't showing progression in the program have sufficient information from the WBA to help them recognize and address their shortcomings. It is also important to assure that mechanisms exist to provide understanding about how, and how much, learners use WBA information. For example, surveys or focus groups with learners and/or their supervising coaches or mentors can reveal how learners approach the responsibility of collecting WBAs and how they use WBA information to guide their future learning.

Monitoring for Bias

Despite the many benefits of WBAs as a form of learner assessment, their use is not without challenges. To ensure equity in assessment, implementers must address bias. Because WBAs are a form of judgment by a supervisor of a learner, undesirable bias can influence those judgments. Just as implicit bias influences clinicians' interactions with patients, implicit

Case 5-4: WBA to Enhance Feedback about Communication and Professionalism

Problem:

In a postgraduate medical education program, a competence committee identifies concerns about some residents' communication skills and professionalism. Members of the committee review data from end-of-month global evaluations and results from a new ambulatory general practice clinic patient satisfaction survey. On a mailed survey, patients rate some resident physicians below the expected benchmark for communication and timely follow-up. Committee members also share comments during the competency committee meeting that reflect some concerns about residents' professionalism not being captured by the end-of-month global evaluations.

Solution:

Residents need feedback about their communication skills with patients and their management of patient care needs both during and between clinical visits. Preceptors need a tool to evaluate residents' communication and professionalism that guides them to discuss formative feedback and provide needed information for the competence committee. To gather additional information from other sources for incorporation into the competence committee workflow and feedback for learners, the program adopts a WBA tool for preceptors to give feedback on patient communication and professionalism during patient visits and provision of follow-up care outside of clinic visits. The program also initiates a patient-satisfaction survey with ratings and narrative comments. Handouts in the waiting room educate patients about their role in contributing to residents' education. Faculty and residents receive training about expectations for achievement of competence in all competencies relevant to ambulatory care.

Take Home Message:

Residents place increased emphasis on building their communication skills with patients. Care outside of visits increases and patient satisfaction improves. Multisource feedback proves to be valuable to support feedback dialogues between learners and supervisors within a competency-based medical education program.

bias influences clinicians' interactions with and inferences about learners. Evidence of bias in assessment of learners exists using a variety of assessment tools. For example, group differences manifest in quantitative ratings of learners based on learner gender and race or ethnicity [49]. Similarly, there are group differences in narrative comments describing learner performance based on learner gender or race or ethnicity [50,51]. Small differences in assessed performance can lead to larger differences in subsequent grades and awards [52].

Therefore, a robust implementation of WBA must include strategies to acknowledge and reduce the risk of bias and engage in ongoing monitoring for bias. A first step is to educate assessors about the risk of bias in learner assessment. To achieve broad participation and awareness about the risk of bias and strategies to mitigate harmful bias in the process of learner assessment requires an institutional approach to this education. A variety of educational formats have been proposed, such as having assessors undergo the implicit association test or participate in discussion or workshops about bias [53]. At the institutional level, commitment to ongoing monitoring of collected learner assessment data enables identification of any group differences in performance ratings or comments that could signal bias.

Case 5-5 provides strategies for programs to monitor their data for group differences in performance that can signal inequity or bias. These data enhance transparency and direct interventions such as faculty development and creation of a microaggressions reporting system that enables program improvement for equity.

Ethical Issues

From an ethical perspective, assessment of performance should be fair and equitable, and WBA implementation that follows best practices in assessment can successfully fulfill multiple ethical principles in service to justice. For example, learners must understand the predefined criteria on which their performance will be assessed to achieve truthfulness as well as transparency in the process. Expectations should be clear about when and how WBA should be conducted and how the information will be used for formative or summative assessment and ensure that learners and their educators have mutual understanding about this process (again creating truthfulness). Learners' opportunity to drive some WBA encounters and receive detailed feedback engages them in the process to provide both

Case 5-5: Bias and Microaggressions: Monitoring and Quality Assurance

Problem:

A supervisor commits a microaggression by making a culturally insensitive comment about a patient in front of the team, whose members include a student from a group underrepresented in medicine. For the student, the comment sticks and interferes with his performance when giving a case presentation and working with peers. However, he does not discuss this situation with either the resident or his clerkship advisor. The supervisor rates this learner poorly as a consequence.

Solution:

To achieve assessment, including WBA, that avoids harmful bias and discrimination, faculty engage in training about working with and assessing diverse learners. Required training in diversity, equity, and inclusion for faculty supervisors includes the Implicit Association Test and a facilitated workshop. Program leaders introduce a new confidential reporting system for issues of perceived bias so that the learning environment is monitored and interventions are possible for individuals or settings in which bias arises. Program evaluators monitor for bias in assessment information as part of quality assurance. Annual review and reporting of WBA data for the group of learners and observers provides transparency and identifies any population group differences based on gender, race, or ethnicity.

Take Home Message:

To achieve equity in assessment, differences in scores based on gender, race, or ethnicity are identified, along with a few examples of written WBA comments that include inappropriate comments about learners' gender, race, or ethnicity. These examples are shared with learners and faculty. A reporting system for learners to report problems such as microaggressions in the learning environment is created. With ongoing training and data monitoring, group differences in learners' assessed performance decreases. This issue is further addressed in Chapter 8.

autonomy and beneficence. Training for assessors about mitigating bias reduces the risk of group differences in ratings of performance in order to ensure nonmaleficence.

▌ CONCLUSION

This chapter has presented key information for implementation of WBA within a program of assessment. Commitment to the purposes of WBA among all stakeholders as a tool to promote feedback to learners and monitor their progressive achievement of competence is foundational to successful use. Implementation considerations address the importance of culture change through a robust and ongoing communication strategy. Careful tool selection aligns with the aims of WBA to generate rich data about learners. The process of data aggregation, using technology, facilitates group decision-making about learners' progress within the program. Quality assurance with WBA entails ongoing process and data review through implementation and data monitoring, assessor training rather than a sole focus on assessment tools, providing feedback to assessors, and monitoring learner's outcomes to ensure validity of decision-making about learner progress.

▌ REFERENCES

1. Swanwick T, Chana N. Workplace-Based Assessment. *British Journal of Hospital Medicine*. 2009;70(5):290–293. doi:10.12968/hmed.2009.70.5.42235
2. Miller GE. The Assessment of Clinical Skills/Competence/Performance. *Acad Med*. 1990;65(9 Suppl):S63–S67. doi:10.1097/00001888-199009000-00045
3. Norcini JJ. ABC of Learning and Teaching in Medicine: Work Based Assessment. *BMJ*. 2003;326(7392):753–755. doi:10.1136/bmj.326.7392.753
4. van der Vleuten CPM, Schuwirth LWT, Driessen EW, et al. A Model for Programmatic Assessment Fit for Purpose. *Med Teach*. 2012;34(3):205–214. doi:10.3109/0142159X.2012.652239
5. Watling CJ, Ajjawi R, Bearman M. Approaching Culture in Medical Education: Three Perspectives. *Med Educ*. 2020;54(4):289–295. doi:10.1111/medu.14037
6. Kotter JP. *Leading Change*. Cambridge, MA: Harvard Business Press; 1996.
7. Norcini J, Burch V. Workplace-Based Assessment as an Educational Tool—AMEE Guide No. 31. *Med Teach*. 2007;29(9):855–871. doi:10.1080/01421590701775453
8. Bok HGJ, Teunissen PW, Favier RP, et al. Programmatic Assessment of Competency-Based Workplace Learning: When Theory Meets Practice. *BMC Med Educ*. 2013;13:123. doi:10.1186/1472-6920-13-123

9. Heeneman S, Oudkerk Pool A, Schuwirth LWT, van der Vleuten CPM, Driessen EW. The Impact of Programmatic Assessment on Student Learning: Theory versus Practice. *Med Educ*. 2015;49(5):487–498. doi:10.1111/medu.12645

10. Al-Kadri HM, Al-Kadi MT, Van Der Vleuten CPM. Workplace-Based Assessment and Students' Approaches to Learning: A Qualitative Inquiry. *Med Teach*. 2013;35(Suppl 1):S31–S38. doi:10.3109/0142159X.2013.765547

11. Govaerts MJB, van der Vleuten CPM, Holmboe ES. Managing Tensions in Assessment: Moving Beyond Either–Or Thinking. *Med Educ*. 2019;53(1):64–75. doi:10.1111/medu.13656

12. Kogan JR, Hess BJ, Conforti LN, Holmboe ES. What Drives Faculty Ratings of Residents' Clinical Skills? The Impact of Faculty's Own Clinical Skills. *Acad Med*. 2010;85(10 Suppl):S25–S28. doi:10.1097/ACM.0b013e3181ed1aa3

13. Watling C, LaDonna KA, Lingard L, Voyer S, Hatala R. "Sometimes the Work Just Needs to Be Done": Socio-Cultural Influences on Direct Observation in Medical Training. *Medical Education*. 2016;50(10):1054–1064. doi:10.1111/medu.13062

14. Molloy E, Boud D. Seeking a Different Angle on Feedback in Clinical Education: The Learner as Seeker, Judge and User of Performance Information. *Med Educ*. 2013;47(3):227–229. doi:10.1111/medu.12116

15. Telio S, Regehr G, Ajjawi R. Feedback and the Educational Alliance: Examining Credibility Judgments and Their Consequences. *Med Educ*. 2016;50(9):933–942. doi:10.1111/medu.13063

16. Watling CJ, Ginsburg S. Assessment, Feedback and the Alchemy of Learning. *Med Educ*. 2019;53(1):76–85. doi:10.1111/medu.13645

17. Sargeant J, Lockyer J, Mann K, et al. Facilitated Reflective Performance Feedback: Developing an Evidence- and Theory-Based Model That Builds Relationship, Explores Reactions and Content, and Coaches for Performance Change (R2C2). *Acad Med*. 2015;90(12):1698–1706. doi:10.1097/ACM.0000000000000809

18. Dweck C. What Having a "Growth Mindset" Actually Means. *Harvard Business Review*. Published online January 13, 2016:1–5.

19. Ramani S, Könings KD, Mann KV, Pisarski EE, van der Vleuten CPM. About Politeness, Face, and Feedback: Exploring Resident and Faculty Perceptions of How Institutional Feedback Culture Influences Feedback Practices. *Acad Med*. 2018;93(9):1348–1358. doi:10.1097/ACM.0000000000002193

20. Lave J, Wenger E. *Situated Learning: Legitimate Peripheral Participation*. Cambridge, England: Cambridge University Press; 1991.

21. *Politeness: Some Universals in Language Usage*. Reissue edition. Cambridge, England: Cambridge University Press; 1987.

22. Jelovsek JE, Kow N, Diwadkar GB. Tools for the Direct Observation and Assessment of Psychomotor Skills in Medical Trainees: A Systematic Review. *Medical Education*. 2013;47(7):650–673. doi:10.1111/medu.12220

23. Kogan JR, Holmboe ES, Hauer KE. Tools for Direct Observation and Assessment of Clinical Skills Of Medical Trainees: A Systematic Review. *JAMA*. 2009;302(12):1316–1326. doi:10.1001/jama.2009.1365

24. Eva KW. On the Generality of Specificity. *Medical Education*. 2003;37(7):587–588. doi:10.1046/j.1365-2923.2003.01563.x

25. Moonen-van Loon JMW, Overeem K, Donkers HHLM, van der Vleuten CPM, Driessen EW. Composite Reliability of a Workplace-Based Assessment Toolbox for Postgraduate Medical Education. *Advances in Health Sciences Education*. 2013;18(5):1087–1102. doi:10.1007/s10459-013-9450-z

26. Jong LH de, Bok HGJ, Kremer WDJ, Vleuten CPM van der. Programmatic Assessment: Can We Provide Evidence for Saturation of Information? *Medical Teacher*. 2019;41(6):678–682. doi:10.1080/0142159X.2018.1555369

27. Govaerts M, van der Vleuten CPM. Validity in Work-Based Assessment: Expanding Our Horizons. *Med Educ*. 2013;47(12):1164–1174. doi:10.1111/medu.12289

28. van der Vleuten CPM, Schuwirth LWT. Assessing Professional Competence: From Methods to Programmes. *Med Educ*. 2005;39(3):309–317. doi:10.1111/j.1365-2929.2005.02094.x

29. Norcini J, Anderson B, Bollela V, et al. Criteria for Good Assessment: Consensus Statement and Recommendations from the Ottawa 2010 Conference. *Med Teach*. 2011;33(3):206–214. doi:10.3109/0142159X.2011.551559

30. Pelgrim EM, Kramer AWM, Mokkink HGA, et al. In-Training Assessment Using Direct Observation of Single-Patient Encounters: A Literature Review. *Adv Health Sci Educ Theory Pract*. 2011;16(1):131–142. doi:10.1007/s10459-010-9235-6

31. Duijn CCMA, Dijk EJ van, Mandoki M, Bok HGJ, Cate OTJT. Assessment Tools for Feedback and Entrustment Decisions in the Clinical Workplace: A Systematic Review. *J Vet Med Educ*. 2019;46(3):340–352. doi:10.3138/jvme.0917-123r

32. Norcini J, Anderson MB, Bollela V, et al. 2018 Consensus Framework for Good Assessment. *Medical Teacher*. 2018;0(0):1-8. doi:10.1080/0142159X.2018.1500016

33. Downing SM. Threats to the Validity of Clinical Teaching Assessments: What About Rater Error? *Med Educ*. 2005;39(4):353–355. doi:10.1111/j.1365-2929.2005.02138.x

34. Gingerich A, Kogan J, Yeates P, Govaerts M, Holmboe E. Seeing the "Black Box" Differently: Assessor Cognition from Three Research Perspectives. *Med Educ*. 2014;48(11):1055–1068. doi:10.1111/medu.12546

35. Kurtz SM, Silverman JD. The Calgary–Cambridge Referenced Observation Guides: An Aid to Defining the Curriculum and Organizing the Teaching in Communication Training Programmes. *Medical Education*. 1996;30(2):83–89. doi:10.1111/j.1365–2923.1996.tb00724.x

36. Makoul G. The SEGUE Framework for Teaching and Assessing Communication Skills. *Patient Educ Couns*. 2001;45(1):23–34. doi:10.1016/s0738-3991(01)00136-7

37. Lörwald AC, Lahner F-M, Mooser B, et al. Influences on the Implementation of Mini-CEX and DOPS for Postgraduate Medical Trainees' Learning: A Grounded Theory Study. *Medical Teacher*. 2019;41(4):448–456. doi:10.1080/0142159X.2018.1497784

38. Watling C, Driessen E, van der Vleuten CPM, Lingard L. Learning Culture and Feedback: An International Study of Medical Athletes and Musicians. *Med Educ.* 2014;48(7):713–723. doi:10.1111/medu.12407

39. Bates J, Konkin J, Suddards C, Dobson S, Pratt D. Student Perceptions of Assessment and Feedback in Longitudinal Integrated Clerkships. *Med Educ.* 2013;47(4):362–374. doi:10.1111/medu.12087

40. Kogan JR, Hatala R, Hauer KE, Holmboe E. Guidelines: The Do's, Don'ts and Don't Knows of Direct Observation of Clinical Skills in Medical Education. *Perspect Med Educ.* 2017;6(5):286–305. doi:10.1007/s40037-017-0376-7

41. Lefroy J, Watling C, Teunissen PW, Brand P. Guidelines: The Do's, Don'ts and Don't Knows of Feedback for Clinical Education. *Perspect Med Educ.* 2015;4(6):284–299. doi:10.1007/s40037-015-0231-7

42. Arnstead N, Campisi P, Takahashi SG, et al. Feedback Frequency in Competence by Design: A Quality Improvement Initiative. *J Grad Med Educ.* 2020;12(1):46–50. doi:10.4300/JGME-D-19-00358.1

43. London M, Smither JW. Feedback Orientation, Feedback Culture, and the Longitudinal Performance Management Process. *Human Resource Management Review.* 2002;12(1):81–100. doi:10.1016/S1053-4822(01)00043-2

44. Schuwirth LWT, Van der Vleuten CPM. Programmatic Assessment: From Assessment of Learning to Assessment for Learning. *Med Teach.* 2011;33(6):478–485. doi:10.3109/0142159X.2011.565828

45. Boscardin C, Fergus KB, Hellevig B, Hauer KE. Twelve Tips to Promote Successful Development of a Learner Performance Dashboard within a Medical Education Program. *Medical Teacher.* 2017;0(0):1–7. doi:10.1080/0142159X.2017.1396306

46. Chan T, Sebok-Syer S, Thoma B, et al. Learning Analytics in Medical Education Assessment: The Past, the Present, and the Future. *AEM Educ Train.* 2018;2(2):178–187. doi:10.1002/aet2.10087

47. Andolsek K, Padmore J, Hauer KE, Ekpenyong A, Edgar L, Holmboe E. Clinical Competency Committees. A Guidebook for Programs, 3rd Ed. https://www.acgme.org/Portals/0/ACGMEClinicalCompetencyCommitteeGuidebook.pdf

48. Frank AK, O'Sullivan P, Mills LM, Muller-Juge V, Hauer KE. Clerkship Grading Committees: The Impact of Group Decision-Making for Clerkship Grading. *J Gen Intern Med.* 2019;34(5):669–676. doi:10.1007/s11606-019-04879-x

49. Dayal A, O'Connor DM, Qadri U, Arora VM. Comparison of Male vs Female Resident Milestone Evaluations by Faculty During Emergency Medicine Residency Training. *JAMA Intern Med.* 2017;177(5):651–657. doi:10.1001/jamainternmed.2016.9616

50. Mueller AS, Jenkins TM, Osborne M, et al. Gender Differences in Attending Physicians' Feedback to Residents: A Qualitative Analysis. *J Grad Med Educ.* 2017;9(5):577–585. doi:10.4300/JGME-D-17-00126.1

51. Rojek AE, Khanna R, Yim JWL, et al. Differences in Narrative Language in Evaluations of Medical Students by Gender and Under-Represented Minority Status. *J Gen Intern Med*. 2019;34(5):684–691. doi:10.1007/s11606-019-04889-9

52. Teherani A, Hauer KE, Fernandez A, King TE, Lucey C. How Small Differences in Assessed Clinical Performance Amplify to Large Differences in Grades and Awards: A Cascade with Serious Consequences for Students Underrepresented in Medicine. *Acad Med*. 2018;93(9):1286–1292. doi:10.1097/ACM.0000000000002323

53. Karpinski A, Hilton JL. Attitudes and the Implicit Association Test. *Journal of Personality and Social Psychology*. 2001;81(5):774–788. doi:10.1037/0022-3514.81.5.774

Quality Assurance in Programmatic Assessment

6

Lubberta H. de Jong, Harold G.J. Bok, Beth S. Bierer, and
Cees P.M. van der Vleuten

CHAPTER HIGHLIGHTS

- Programmatic assessment aims to align assessment to modern education approaches.
- Programmatic assessment can have multiple designs. In this chapter, three different implementations within the health professions education are presented.
- Quality assurance within a programmatic approach to assessment is multifaceted.

▌ ORIENTATION TO THE CHAPTER

Over the last decade, programmatic assessment has gained popularity in health professions education. This modern approach requires new ways of thinking about assessment. Programmatic assessment provides a framework to guide assessment practices, which allows health professions institutes to design their programs optimally for their (educational) contexts. This also means there is no one-size-fits-all implementation of programmatic assessment. The same holds true for quality assurance processes involved in programmatic assessment. In this chapter, the principles and rationale of programmatic assessment are outlined and then followed by three cases with varying implementations. Informed by experiences from practice and the literature, in the last section of this chapter the authors discuss implications for quality assurance through the presentation of overarching themes.

INTRODUCTION—PRINCIPLES OF PROGRAMMATIC ASSESSMENT

A conventional approach to assessment is a modular summative approach. Modules of education are completed with an assessment that needs to be passed based on a minimum passing level. Failing means that the student has to repeat the assessment or ultimately the entire course. Once passed, learners move on to the next module and, when all modules are completed, the learner is considered competent. There are many downsides to this summative approach. It leads to test-directed studying and learning for the test, which is often associated with superficial learning styles [1]. Learned information is easily forgotten. There is little information in the assessment. Typically, grades are used. But grades are extremely poor information carriers [2], which is particularly true for the assessment of complex skills. When additional feedback is given, learners are not inclined to use the feedback in a summative assessment system [3] to regulate their performance. Summative systems of assessment often have few longitudinal components that look at the growth of competence. Finally, individual assessments lead to many false positive and negative pass–fail decisions simply because of measurement error and issues of reliability [4]. The summative approach to assessment is poorly constructively aligned to more modern approaches to learning. Modern approaches to learning are competency-based [5,6]. Competency-based medical education focuses on complex competencies in addition to medical knowledge. These competencies are typically behavioral (communication, collaboration, leadership, etc.) and can only be assessed by observation and professional judgment of that observation in a more longitudinal fashion. Modern education approaches emphasize self-directed learning as a basis for lifelong learning. These modern approaches to education are both seen in classroom teaching as well as in workplace-based learning, but also across all levels of education (undergraduate, postgraduate, lifelong learning). Programmatic assessment is an attempt to better constructively align assessment to modern education. It is a system-based approach to assessment [7]. A purposeful design of an assessment program as a whole is usually based on a competency framework or any other overarching structure (e.g., based on entrustable professional activities). Programmatic assessment has several building blocks based on previous research consistencies in assessment [8,9]:

- Every assessment is considered to be a single data point.
- Single data points are optimized for learning, implying that the assessment provides meaningful information to the learners—that is, rich feedback.

- Pass–fail decisions are removed from single data points.
- There is a mix of methods of assessment. The choice of a method depends on the educational justification for using that method at that moment in time and on the relationship with the rest of the assessment program.
- Learner performance is longitudinally monitored by a coach or mentor. Learner and mentor have periodic meetings. In preparation for these meetings, the performance is self-analyzed by the learner. Plans can be made for remediation.
- The summative or formative distinction is replaced by a continuum of stakes. An individual data point is low-stakes.
- A high-stakes decision is taken after a longer period of time (i.e., promotion to the next year of training) based on triangulation of many data points. This is the principle of proportionality. The higher the stakes, the more data points are needed.
- An intermediate-stakes decision is taken before the high-stakes decision (i.e., half-way through the year) to inform the learners about their progress. Learner performance monitoring and an intermediate performance assessment promote self-directed learning and prevent any surprises from occurring in the high-stakes decision moment.

Programmatic assessment has, since its inception [9,10], been implemented both at undergraduate [11,12] and postgraduate level [13,14] of education.

We now present three case studies (**Cases 6-1**, **6-2** and **6-3**) describing different implementations of programmatic assessment. Each case provides a brief description of the current program in general, the rationale for adopting programmatic assessment, key assessment system design features, and quality assurance strategies.

CASE 6-1—CLEVELAND CLINIC LERNER COLLEGE OF MEDICINE (CCLCM)

Program Description

The Cleveland Clinic Lerner College of Medicine (CCLCM) of Case Western Reserve University in Ohio was established in 2004 as a 5-year program to produce physician investigators who would be prepared to advance biomedical research and clinical practice. Each class has 32 graduate-entry students. The curriculum is organized around nine competencies that map to the Accreditation Council for Graduate Medical Education (ACGME) competencies [15] and CCLCM's mission-specific competencies (research and scholarship, personal and professional development, reflective practice) [16,17]. Students complete organ-based courses in years 1 and 2 in tandem with the clinical curriculum, which begins in year 1 with skill-building sessions involving standardized patients and continues in year 2 with advanced communication and physical diagnosis experiences. Students apply clinical skills when having first contact with ambulatory patients in bimonthly (year 1) and weekly (year 2) longitudinal clinics. Students complete clerkships and electives in years 3–5. Research is interspersed throughout two summer research blocks, a weekly year 1–2 seminar series, and year 3–5 research-skill development sessions. Each student devotes 48 weeks in year 4 to complete and defend a hypothesis-driven thesis project. Students do not take summative examinations or receive grades for courses or clerkships. Instead, students create summative portfolios with advisor guidance that provide the basis for high-stakes progression decisions in years 1, 2, and 4.

Reasons for Change

Prominent researchers and expert panels have raised concerns about the declining physician-investigator workforce in the United States [18–21]. In response to this workforce shortage of physician investigators, the Cleveland Clinic's leadership built on the institution's strengths in translational and clinical research to create a new medical school program with a focused research mission. Our overarching goal was to produce graduates who had a passion for scientific inquiry, skills for critical thinking, and broad-based clinical expertise. Our faculty recalled how taking periodic summative examinations as students had not prepared them well for clinical practice. They wanted CCLCM students to become "reflective practitioners" of medicine and science with a drive for lifelong learning, complemented by a critical approach to self-assessment and self-improvement [22].

In being a new school, curriculum planners could design CCLCM's medical school curriculum and unique assessment system *de novo* without the burden of maintaining an existing curriculum at the same time. This flexibility provided curriculum planners with time and resources to consult with experts and craft guiding principles that subsequently informed key design decisions. For instance, problem-based learning was adopted as the instructional approach for the basic science curriculum, given the guiding principle to use active learning methods. Curriculum planners also decided to select assessment methods that emphasized "assessment *for* learning" rather than "assessment *of* learning" [9,10,23]. To help achieve this vision, curriculum planners adopted assessment methods that aligned with programmatic assessment principles [12].

Designed Assessment Program

CCLCM's educational program has several building blocks purposefully designed to encourage students to take personal responsibility for their own learning. The curriculum is organized around nine competencies, with each one having milestones that students can use to gauge their progress and performance. These milestones map directly onto curricular experiences and increase in difficulty as students gain proficiency and experience. As an illustration, Table 6-1 shows the milestones for the research and scholarship competency.

Table 6-1   MILESTONES FOR THE RESEARCH AND SCHOLARSHIP COMPETENCY AT CLEVELAND CLINIC LERNER COLLEGE OF MEDICINE AT DIFFERENT TIME POINTS (YEARS 1, 2, AND 5)

Competency	Year 1	Year 2	Year 5
Research and Scholarship Demonstrates knowledge and skills required to interpret, critically evaluate, and conduct research.	Demonstrates ability to critically review basic science research papers. Generates research hypothesis and articulates a strategy to test that hypothesis. Actively participates in the performance of laboratory procedures and interpretation of information relevant to their basic science research.	Demonstrates ability to critically review clinical research papers. Generates research questions to explore hypotheses in clinical science. Applies principles and skills in medical biostatistics and clinical epidemiology to the analysis of data. Demonstrates understanding of clinical research methods needed to test hypotheses.	Analyzes and effectively critiques a broad range of research papers. Demonstrates ability to generate a research hypothesis and formulate questions to test the hypothesis. Demonstrates ability to initiate, complete and explain all aspects of his or her own research project.

Students receive low-stake feedback from different assessors (e.g., clinical preceptors, problem-based learning (PBL) facilitators, research advisors, peers) across courses and contexts throughout the 5-year program [24]. This feedback is predominately narrative, with assessors documenting students' strengths and improvement areas in relation to observable behaviors listed on assessment forms. Though students complete traditional assessments in years 1–2 for medical knowledge (weekly essay questions and Multiple Choice Questions [MCQs]) and clinical skills (Objective Structured Clinical Examinations [OSCEs]), these assessments remain low-stake [24,25]. All assessments are automatically uploaded into an electronic portfolio (e-portfolio) that students can access easily for timely feedback. This rich, multisource feedback provides the foundation of CCLCM's portfolio-based assessment system. Consequently, both faculty and students receive formal training on how to provide written narrative feedback for competencies.

Each student is assigned a physician advisor (PA) at program entry who serves as the student's feedback coach. PAs meet regularly with their students to help students decode and process assessment feedback, prioritize learning needs, create portfolios, and generate learning plans. PAs also provide reassurance as students adjust to a unique learning environment that requires them to utilize new learning strategies (e.g., preparing for seminars, asking questions, developing learning objective presentations) than those previously used when preparing for episodic summative examinations (e.g., cramming for tests, memorizing notes, attending review sessions) [26,27].

Students generate two types of portfolios during their medical school experience. Students construct formative portfolios during year 1 (three formative portfolios) and year 2 (two formative portfolios) with guidance from their PAs. Formative portfolios require students to review their assessment evidence and reflect on their performance. Students then write portfolio essays for various milestones within each competency, being sure to cite assessment evidence that supports their progress and achievement. This process is analogous to citing evidence in a research paper. PAs review their students' formative portfolios, offering students feedback and advice on how to apply the reflective practice cycle (i.e., identify goals, implement strategies, and monitor performance). Students construct summative portfolios at the end of years 1, 2, and 4. PAs officially attest to the promotion committee that students' summative portfolios accurately represent their students' abilities. Summative portfolios provide the basis for high-stake progression decisions.

The promotion committee is made up of approximately 30 senior clinicians and researchers and is responsible for making progress decisions. This committee begins each summative portfolio review by independently reading and rating four randomly selected portfolios. The committee then meets as a group and uses an audience response system to record competency-specific decisions (met, met with concerns, formal performance improvement, insufficient evidence) and overall performance decisions (met, met with concerns, formal performance improvement, repeat year, dismiss) for "standard-setting" portfolios. Once consensus is achieved, the committee divides into dyads in which each pair reviews three to four summative portfolios. The promotion committee reconvenes to vote on these portfolios. The committee concludes the summative portfolio review process by sending each student a personalized letter documenting the committee's promotion decision as well as commenting on the student's strengths, improvement areas, and reflective abilities.

Periodically, a student may require additional assistance and support. For instance, a student may consistently struggle with meeting deadlines (professionalism) or may infrequently contribute to class discussions (interpersonal and communication skills). The promotion committee ensures that students reflect on performance gaps and develop formal performance improvement plans (FPIP) to address these deficiencies. The promotion committee releases students from their FPIPs when students provide sufficient documentation of achievement. This remediation process remains both student centered and student directed, with positive outcomes in most cases [28].

Quality Assurance

The College Assessment and Outcomes Committee (COAC) oversees all aspects of CCLCM's portfolio-based assessment system. This centralized oversight ensures all policies and practices remain aligned with programmatic assessment principles. The director of assessment and evaluation chairs the COAC, which has a broad membership of curriculum deans, chairs of the physician advisor committee and promotion committee, basic and clinical science faculty, and medical students.

We developed an internal quality assurance plan that maps to our assessment system [29]. Table 6-2 presents current monitoring foci, with most methods designed to promote stakeholder engagement. For instance, medical students provide feedback about portfolio processes, weekly knowledge assessments, and courses using multiple methods (questionnaires, informal feedback meetings, focus groups, and exit interviews). Course directors and curriculum planners receive item analysis reports of weekly self-assessment questions and students' aggregate performance scores on OSCEs. These reports help course directors identify items and cases to revise as well curricular areas requiring improvement. Physician

Table 6-2 BLUEPRINT OF QUALITY ASSURANCE PLAN FOR CCLCM'S ASSESSMENT SYSTEM	
Component	**Evaluation Focus**
Fairness *Policies and procedures meet standards for equity and equality.*	• Stakeholders understand portfolio requirements in advance. • Students have equal opportunities to revise portfolios or receive assistance. • Due process guidelines exist if students appeal unfavorable decisions. • Periodically monitor if relationships exist between performance decisions and student demographics.
Reliability *Mechanisms exist that contribute to credible, high-stake decisions.*	• Assessors receive sufficient training to provide consistent, credible high-stake decisions about student performance. • Sufficient assessment evidence exists, using multiple methods across contexts, to document learners' performance in competency domains.
Validity *Qualified assessments make accurate, defensible decisions about learner competence.*	• Curricular experiences and assessment evidence align closely with performance expectations stated in milestones and competencies. • Assessors provide specific feedback to document learners' competence. • Portfolio evidence represents each student's progress and performance. • Assessment evidence provides meaningful, accurate, and timely documentation of learners' competence.
Effects *Assessment system nurtures reflective practice.*	• Students' portfolios present strengths, weaknesses, and reflection in relation to performance of competencies. • Students develop learning plans with physician advisor guidance. • Participants are satisfied with formative and summative portfolio processes. • Participants believe portfolio assessment process contributes to learning.

(continued)

Table 6-2 BLUEPRINT OF QUALITY ASSURANCE PLAN FOR CCLCM'S ASSESSMENT SYSTEM (*CONTINUED*)	
Component	**Evaluation Focus**
Outcomes *Intended and* *unintended* *consequences are* *monitored.*	• Key faculty have adequate time to perform assessment roles in program. • Students and faculty have positive perceptions of learning environment. • Monitor student performance on licensure exams (USMLE Step 1 and USMLE Step 2 CK) for unintended outcomes. • Monitor if assessment system places students at a disadvantage when applying for residency programs. • Monitor forces that may undermine the "assessment *for* learning" culture.

advisors regularly review students' assessment evidence and notify the director of assessment and evaluation of any problems (e.g., missing assessments). Promotion committee members debrief after each summative portfolio review and provide feedback about the assessment system (e.g., clarity of milestones, quality and quantity of assessment evidence, curricular strengths, etc.).

The director of assessment and evaluation generates an annual report summarizing the assessment system's strengths, weaknesses, and noteworthy changes and offers recommendations for the coming year to the CAOC and curriculum steering committee, the oversight group for the overall educational program. This internal reporting provides opportunities to review and discuss the assessment system as a whole with a variety of stakeholders.

CCLCM made faculty development a quality assurance priority. Physician advisors meet weekly as a committee to discuss student performance and assessment issues that may present during the academic year. These weekly meetings provide a community of practice for advisors to share strategies with one another or seek informal advice from experienced PAs. Each new PA receives formal training about performance expectations and curriculum components. Promotion committee members meet monthly. New promotion committee members undergo formal training to orient them to the portfolio review process and curriculum. The entire promotion committee engages in some form of faculty development (e.g., promotion letter writing and curriculum updates) before each summative portfolio review. Faculty assessors who serve in critical assessment roles such as PBL facilitators and longitudinal preceptors must participate in faculty development. PBL facilitators, for instance, receive coaching regarding the specificity and appropriateness of their narrative written feedback to students. Unfortunately, the quality and quantity of narrative feedback students receive during core clerkships, electives, and acting internships drops considerably in years 3–5. We recently implemented a longitudinal integrated clerkship at the Cleveland Clinic where CCLCM students spend dedicated time with a core group of clinical preceptors at one site. We hope that providing continuity through a trained cadre of faculty assessors will improve the feedback students receive during clinical experiences.

Our assessment system is externally reviewed every eight years by the Liaison Committee on Medical Education (LCME), the accrediting body for all North American allopathic medical schools. We monitor LCME accreditation standards related to assessment and the overall educational program in collaboration with Case Western Reserve University. CCLCM is currently a fully accredited medical school program. Our next LCME accreditation will occur during 2024–2025.

Lessons Learned

We gleaned several lessons by using a purposeful approach to monitor and improve our portfolio-based assessment system. The foundation of our assessment system rests on the quality and quantity of assessment feedback that students receive from different assessors across contexts. Students must have timely, specific, and sufficient feedback for all competencies and milestones to become empowered to self-assess their performance and implement improvement plans [24,26,27]. Formative and summative portfolios are tools within the assessment system designed to have students review their assessment evidence and reflect on their performance. Physician advisors play a pivotal role in helping students navigate the assessment system. They also verify that summative portfolios accurately represent students' performance, thereby enhancing the trustworthiness of student-constructed portfolios. Promotion committee members must know the curriculum and available assessment evidence to make informed progression decisions. In addition, both faculty and students need training and encouragement on how to provide and receive specific narrative feedback to support learning, especially because most at our institution are more familiar with traditional, summative assessment described previously in this chapter. Consequently, we recommend having ongoing dialogue with students, faculty, and other stakeholders to help foster and sustain an "assessment *for* learning" culture.

CASE 6-2—MAASTRICHT UNIVERSITY PHYSICIAN CLINICAL INVESTIGATOR PROGRAM (PCI)

Program Description

The Physician Clinical Investigator (PCI) program is a graduate-entry program of 4 years. Fifty students are selected after completing a relevant biomedical bachelor's program. In addition to their medical degree, they receive a master's of clinical research on graduation. One year in total across the 4 years is consumed on this research capacity development. The Netherlands has adopted the CanMEDS framework on a national basis [30]. The program is competency-based. The first year is problem based in the classical sense. Learners work in tutorials groups of 10 under the guidance of a tutor. The starting point is a written clinical problem. There is an elaborate clinical skills training program synchronized by content. Other practicals and a few lectures may be given. In the second year, the paper cases are replaced by real patients [31]. In the tutorial group, a clinical case is prepared. Learners then go in pairs to the outpatient clinic where a real patient has been selected by a clinician. One learner will see the patient while the other and the clinician observe. The other learner will attend the patient the next time. After the learners have seen the patient, they receive feedback. Then learning objectives are being formulated and the normal problem-based cycle of self-study and reporting is being completed. The third year consists of clinical rotations. The fourth year consists of roughly half a year of research and half a year of a clinical rotation of the learner's preference. The topic of the research and the rotation may be aligned, all depending on the preferences of the learner. After graduation, they have to complete a postgraduate training program to practice medicine. The Netherlands has no national licensing examinations. Schools themselves are responsible for the quality of their graduates. There is a rigorous accreditation system every 6 years.

Reasons for Change

Maastricht University has a tradition of innovation in education. It started as a new university with undergraduate medicine as the first program in 1974 and adopted problem-based learning for the entire university, which now consists of six faculties (approximately 18,000 students). Self-directed learning is strongly emphasized. The undergraduate 6-year program in medicine has an intake of 340 students per year who gain admission directly from secondary school. The instructional format is problem-based learning. However, the assessment system was rather classic with a large emphasis on end-of-unit exams. These exams had a strong impact on the way learners learned. Despite the emphasis on self-directed learning, there was a strong test orientation [32]. A strong motivation to start the PCI program in 2010 was the desire to innovate further. Innovation would be easier with smaller cohorts. Successful innovations from the graduate-entry program are intended to be upscaled to the undergraduate program. This also holds for programmatic assessment. It was designed first in the graduate-entry PCI program, and programmatic assessment is now also implemented in the master's phase (3-year clinical phase) of the undergraduate medicine program. An implementation in the bachelor's phase has partially been completed (in the clinical skills program), and a full implementation is planned.

Designed Assessment Program

The curriculum is structured in units and internships. In the preclinical program, we have unit-related assessments. They are related to the content of the units, and many of them are single-best-answer tests. Some use open-ended questions. Written assignments require scientific writing. Some units have spaced assessment, with a small assessment every 2 weeks of an 8-week unit. Next to the unit assessments, the program has longitudinal assessment in the cognitive domain and in the noncognitive domain. In the cognitive domain a progress test is used [33]. The progress test is a comprehensive written assessment using mostly scenario-based MCQs. There is a fixed, two-dimensional blueprint of (organ) system categories and disciplines. The progress test is administered every 3 months (4 times per year) to all the students in the curriculum. For every test, new test items are created. A question may be answered by the student or completed with a "I don't know" option. A system of formula scoring is used [34] in which incorrect items are penalized, and the "I don't know" option is scored neutral. The test is developed and administered in collaboration with a total of six of the eight medical schools in the country [35]. Progress testing promotes self-directed learning. It is impossible to study for the test itself. Anything can and will be asked. When learners work and learn regularly, they will find themselves growing automatically. They do not need to cram; they do not need to be anxious. On top of that, the learner gets ample feedback. Every 3 months, a full "X-ray" is being made from the learner's knowledge and can be compared to previous progress tests to monitor growth. Through the multi-institutional approach, each medical school can see how they perform relative to each other. The current progress test is still a paper-and-pencil test. A system of adaptive progress tests has been developed. In an adaptive progress test, every next question for an individual learner is purposefully chosen from a bank of questions and based on the performance on previous items [36]. This approach will allow us to have more flexible online progress test assessments within a few years. The nonparticipating schools in the collaboration will then join the consortium. We will then have a "national knowledge exam" that is highly educationally relevant to learners and faculty and completely owned by the schools. A situation that has been described as a utopia and as an alternative to national end-of curriculum licensing examinations [37].

Within the noncognitive domain in the preclinical years, we rely heavily on peer and tutor assessment and focus on professional behavior assessment. This is done twice during a unit; it is also done multiple times in a communication group in which the students meet each other the whole year and regularly practice clinical skills with simulated patients [38]. Students' professional behavior is evaluated against dealing with your tasks, with others, and with yourself [39]. The forms we use are open for ample narrative feedback. Clinical skills are observed by clinical skills teachers when the learners ask for that, and an observation and a feedback session is held. We hardly have any OSCEs anymore. In the clinical years, we have an elaborate system of Workplace Based Assessment (WBA) consisting of field notes, Mini-Clinical Evaluation Exercises (mini-CEXs), Objective Structured Assessment of Technical Skills (OSATS), and multisource feedback.

All assessment is low-stake. We facilitate feedback with the use of information technology support. Figure 6-1 gives an example of an online system that provides the longitudinal scores on progress testing for an individual learner (the dotted line). The learner can compare the individual performance with the whole of the group. This can also be done for any subscore (disciplines, organ system categories).

All data points are gathered in an e-portfolio that can provide all kinds of aggregation functions. Figure 6-2 shows how a spider chart is made with the individual learner score relative to cohort scores.

A highly useful function of the e-portfolio is that an aggregate of all narrative data can be generated that can also be filtered per competency. It is easy to quickly get an impression of the performance of an individual student. All kinds of other data can be stored as well (reflection reports, assignment outcomes, patient reports) or anything else that may serve as a data point.

Every learner has a mentor who monitors the performance of the students. Each mentor follows the learner throughout the whole program. Every mentor has about 10 learners to guide. Mentors and learners have periodic meetings.

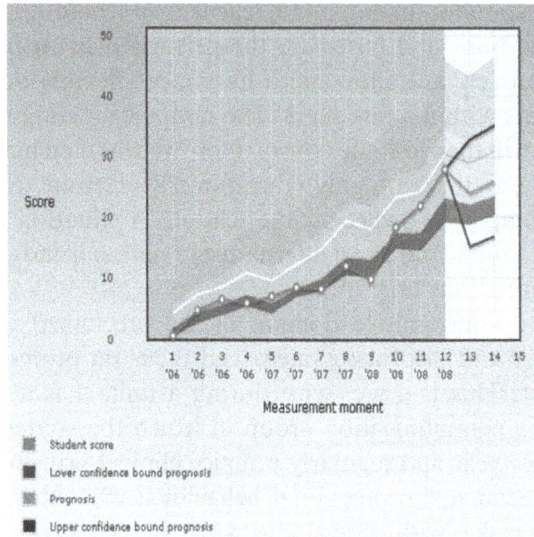

Figure 6-1 • Online longitudinal progress report of an individual learner for 12 tests compared to cohort performance. Measurement moments 13 and 14 are predictions of future scores based on past performance.

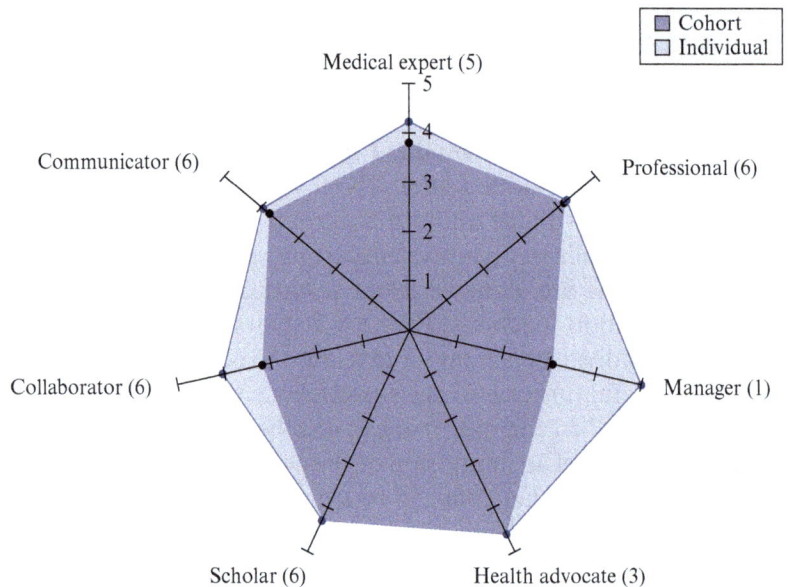

Figure 6-2 • Spider chart of an individual learner's score aggregated across all data points and expressed relative to cohort performance. The bracketed number represent the number of data points.

Progression to the next year is a high-stakes decision moment. The decision is made by a portfolio assessment committee. The mentor provides a recommendation to the committee that may be annotated by the learner, although only the committee decides on a pass–fail basis. Halfway through the year, an intermediate assessment is done. The e-portfolio is judged by another mentor apart from the learner's own mentor, and feedback is given.

Quality Assurance

The QA of the whole program is monitored through several sources. Maastricht University has an elaborate system of internal quality assurance [40]. Every educational activity is systematically evaluated, usually through evaluations from students. When there is a particular concern, qualitative evaluations may be gathered through interviews or evaluation panels. The evaluation includes the assessment. The examination committee is responsible for the quality of the assessment program. Every unit coordinator must submit an assessment plan to the committee and get approval. For standardized testing review, committees review items on quality before test administration. The students are part of the quality assurance system as well. After each test administration, students get copies of their test, the correct answers, and literature references in some cases. The students are given a few days to critique the items. Psychometric information and the student comments are reviewed again by the review committee. Items are dropped as a result of this review, and final scores are being calculated and students receive feedback reports. There is strong commitment to quality control before and after the test in which the learners take part in the quality cycle.

High-stake decisions are based on many data points. All credit points are given for an entire year of training. The high-stakes decision-making is done by a group of experts in an assessment committee. The committee judges individual portfolios using a set of milestones for each competency. A milestone is a narrative description on a competency that describes the expected level at a certain point in time in the curriculum, which is similar to the CCLCM implementation (previous case). The size of the committee varies but usually is around 8–12 members. Assessors are trained for their role. The robustness of the high-stakes decisions is not achieved in a classical way (strict criteria, structured procedures, inter-rater reliability). The robustness is defined as the trustworthiness of the decision-making. Trustworthiness stems from qualitative research. Just like quantitative research, qualitative has a set of criteria and strategies for meeting those criteria [8,41]. Table 6-3 provides an overview of strategies, criteria, assessment strategies, and examples of what we do in our training program [8].

Table 6-3   QUALITATIVE RESEARCH STRATEGIES AND CRITERIA AND SOME EXAMPLES OF ASSESSMENT STRATEGIES FOR BUILDING TRUSTWORTHINESS IN ASSESSMENT DECISIONS

Strategies to Establish Trustworthiness	Criterion	Assessment Strategy	Examples of Strategies Used in the Program
Credibility	Prolonged engagement	• Training of assessors. • The persons who know the student the best (a coach, peers) provide information for the assessment. • Incorporate intermittent feedback cycles in the procedure.	• Elaborate system of faculty development for giving feedback • Intermediate assessment halfway by another mentor • Recommendation by mentor to assessment committee
	Triangulation	• Many assessors should be involved, and different credible groups should be included. • Use multiple sources of assessment within or across methods. • Organize a sequential judgment procedure in which conflicting information necessitates the gathering of more information.	• Large numbers of data points are assembled in portfolio • Mix of modular and longitudinal methods
	Peer examination or peer debriefing	• Organize discussion between assessors (before and intermediate) for benchmarking and discussion of the process and the results. • Separate multiple roles of the assessors by removing the summative assessment decisions from the coaching role.	• Long deliberation on a few learners that require attention • Mentors have no say in the high-stakes decision

	Member checking	Incorporate the learner's point of view in the assessment procedure.	• Learner's may annotate the recommendation given by the mentor • Intermediate assessment by another mentor
	Structural coherence	Organize assessment committee to discuss inconsistencies in the assessment data.	• Committee deliberations proportional to the clarity of information in the portfolio
Transferability	Time sampling	Sample broadly over different contexts and patients.	• Many data points from educational contexts
	Thick description (or dense description)	Incorporate in the assessment instruments possibilities to give qualitative, narrative information. Give narrative information a lot of weight in the assessment procedure.	• All data is captured in e-portfolio • e-portfolio is structured in such a way that allows quick impression formation
Dependability	Stepwise replication	Broad sampling over different assessors.	• Many different assessors are involved in many different educational contexts
Confirmability	Audit	Document the different steps in the assessment process (a formal assessment plan approved by an examination committee, overviews of the results per phase). Organize quality assessment procedures with external auditor. Give learners the possibility to appeal to the assessment decision.	• Plan approval by examination committee • External panel audit in 5-year cycles of accreditation • Learners are part of the quality control cycle • Appeals are possible (but hardly occur)

Reproduced with permission from Van der Vleuten C, Schuwirth L, Scheele F, Driessen EW, Hodges B. The Assessment of Professional Competence: Building Blocks for Theory Development. *Best Pract Res Cl Ob.* 2010;24(6):703–719.

Every 6 years, an external panel does an external accreditation of the whole program. The panel demands evidence that the institution's graduates meet the standards. With programmatic assessment and the elaborate data set that can be generated for every learner, this is a relatively easy task and quite accepted by the accreditation agency.

Finally, scientific research is part of our QA. Often this research provides clarification on how programmatic assessment functions. For example, low-stake assessments are often seen as high-stakes assessments in the view of the learners. We are doing clarification research [42,43] on why this occurs, giving us insights into how to change the approach. Another example deals with tensions in mentoring students toward self-directed learning [44]. Sometimes the research focuses on the quality of the graduates [45]. This research will continue for quite while in the future. Programmatic assessment is derived from research insights [46], but the model itself needs further underpinning with research on why it may work or not. This resembles the model of design-based research [47] with iterations between a model (programmatic assessment) and empirical data gathering on how the model works.

Lessons Learned

Probably the most important lesson is to constantly and continuously involve stakeholders. To implement and run programmatic assessment requires convincing quite a few people. Stakeholders include your leadership, school committees, learners, teachers, clinical preceptors in many different hospitals, and external committees. To make programmatic assessment work, all the people involved need to understand the model, buy into it, and have the skills and the time to make it work. This is a continuous process. You have to keep on convincing or training your people. It is the people who make it successful or not. That will determine if you can make the change from a conventional summative hurdle program to a system with a culture of feedback and learning with a mindset of growth and development.

CASE 6-3—UTRECHT UNIVERSITY VETERINARY MEDICINE (FVMU)

Program Description

The Faculty of Veterinary Medicine at Utrecht University (FVMU) in the Netherlands offers an undergraduate program with a duration of 6 years that results in a master's degree in veterinary medicine. Each year,

225 students are admitted to the program. The program consists of a pre-clinical phase (years 1–3) followed by a clinical phase (years 4–6). Thus far, the preclinical phase obtains a more traditional approach consisting of modular courses thematically built around the organ systems. The clinical phase is competency-based and designed according to the principles of programmatic assessment and will be discussed further in this section.

At the start of the clinical phase, students choose one of three different disciplines—namely, companion animal health, equine medicine, or farm animal health. Education is organized around clinical rotations in which students learn in the clinical workplace at the university's teaching hospital or at extramural veterinary clinics. Students work side by side with clinical staff and have daily patient encounters. During these patient encounters, the students work under the supervision of a member of the clinical team and receive feedback on their performance. Next to the clinical rotations, students have a smaller portion of other learning activities, including electives and a research internship.

Reasons for Change

In 2009, the start of a big curricular renewal for the clinical phase (years 4–6) created an opportunity to design a new learning and assessment program. A SWOT analysis—strengths, weaknesses, opportunities, and threats—of the previous curriculum was performed to identify several weaknesses of the current clinical curriculum. Issues described were (1) the lack of insight into the longitudinal development of students, (2) the fact that there was no documentation of feedback received on direct performance observations, and (3) the absence of truly fulfilling cycles of reflection and improvement. As a consequence, it was difficult to discriminate between students' clinical performance within and across clinical rotations. Another issue was the insufficient alignment between educational strategies and program outcomes. It seemed that the students were just stepping on and off the clerkship train and jumped through hoops instead of focusing on their longitudinal development toward becoming veterinary professionals. In addressing these issues, we investigated the possibilities of creating a sustainable assessment culture focused on learning. This resulted in the design and implementation of an assessment program based on the model of programmatic assessment. Because of the success of the implementation of programmatic assessment in the clinical program, the preclinical program will be redesigned in the upcoming years toward a programmatic approach.

Designed Assessment Program

During clinical rotations, each student collects feedback using multiple low-stakes WBA tools: mini-CEX, multisource feedback (MSF), and evidence-based case report (EBCR). Each tool is designed to combine quantitative information—that is, milestone descriptors on a 5-point scale (1 = novice, 5 = expert)—together with narrative feedback aiming to enhance student learning. To ensure sufficient assessment data regarding the students' performance, each student is required to collect a minimum number of each WBA tool over a variety of different contexts and different rotations. All WBA tools are aggregated at the competency level. These competencies are described in the VetPro framework, specifically designed for the veterinary professional [48]. The VetPro framework consists of seven competency domains: veterinary expertise, communication, collaboration, entrepreneurship, health and welfare, scholarship, and personal development.

Feedback is provided to the student from different assessor perspectives: supervisors, peer students, patient owners, and supporting staff (e.g., the paraveterinary worker). In providing feedback, the assessor has no knowledge of the previous performance of the student as assessed by other assessors. The received feedback is documented in an e-portfolio. Students search for feedback and are responsible for maintaining their e-portfolio. The e-portfolio is designed specifically for the FVMU program and aggregates both the qualitative and quantitative assessment data in order to visualize the data in a meaningful way. This includes an overview of the minimum requirements of the number of WBA tools and learning analytics, such as a spider chart of the quantitative information mapped for all competencies relative to their peers and graphs showing the student's development over time on a competency (see Figure 6-3).

Subsequent to the frequent and longitudinal collection of low-stakes assessment, the student reflects on the received feedback in personal development plans (PDPs) using the ALACT cycle of Korthagen [49]. To foster reflective and deliberate practice and to monitor performance, each student is assigned a mentor. Students meet with their mentors at least twice a year. During these meetings, mentors discuss students' progress and discuss SMART (specific, measurable, acceptable, realistic, and timely) learning goals for the upcoming period as formulated by students. The role of the mentor is twofold. On the one hand, the mentor guides and monitors the student's performance, focusing on diagnosis and timely remediation of the student, which is formally documented as the intermediate assessment. On the other hand, the mentor

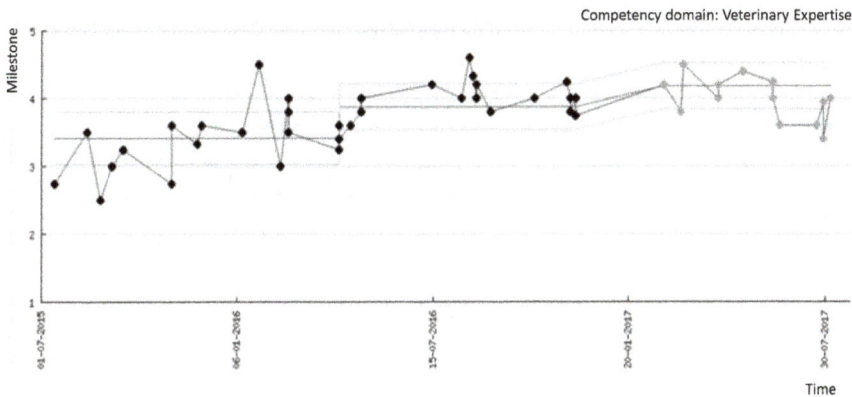

Figure 6-3 • Visualization of the students' longitudinal development as reported in the e-portfolio. The graph shows the milestone development (1–5; *y*-axis) over time (*x*-axis) for the competency veterinary expertise.

is supportive in fostering the student's reflective skills through use of coaching activities.

The preceding process leads to a multitude of low-stakes assessment data points over a longer period of time. After 2 years and after the end of the program, these data points altogether are combined into a high-stakes decision. The high-stakes decision is made by two members of a competency committee. Each assessor independently assesses the portfolio and provides a grade on a scale of 4 to 10 (6 or higher is passing [50]). If there is a significant difference between the two given grades, a third assessor assesses the portfolio. The competency committee meets regularly to discuss difficult portfolios, also serving as calibration sessions.

Figure 6-4 provides a schematic overview of the assessment program at the FVMU [51].

Quality Assurance

The internal quality assurance of the clinical program is performed systematically using the PDCA cycle (plan, do, check, act). Formally, the independent examination committee is responsible for maintaining the quality of the assessment program. Committee members perform frequent internal audits of the procedures in place, the steps taken by the competency committee, and the end products (i.e., e-portfolios) as established by the learners. Together with this, students are actively involved in the quality

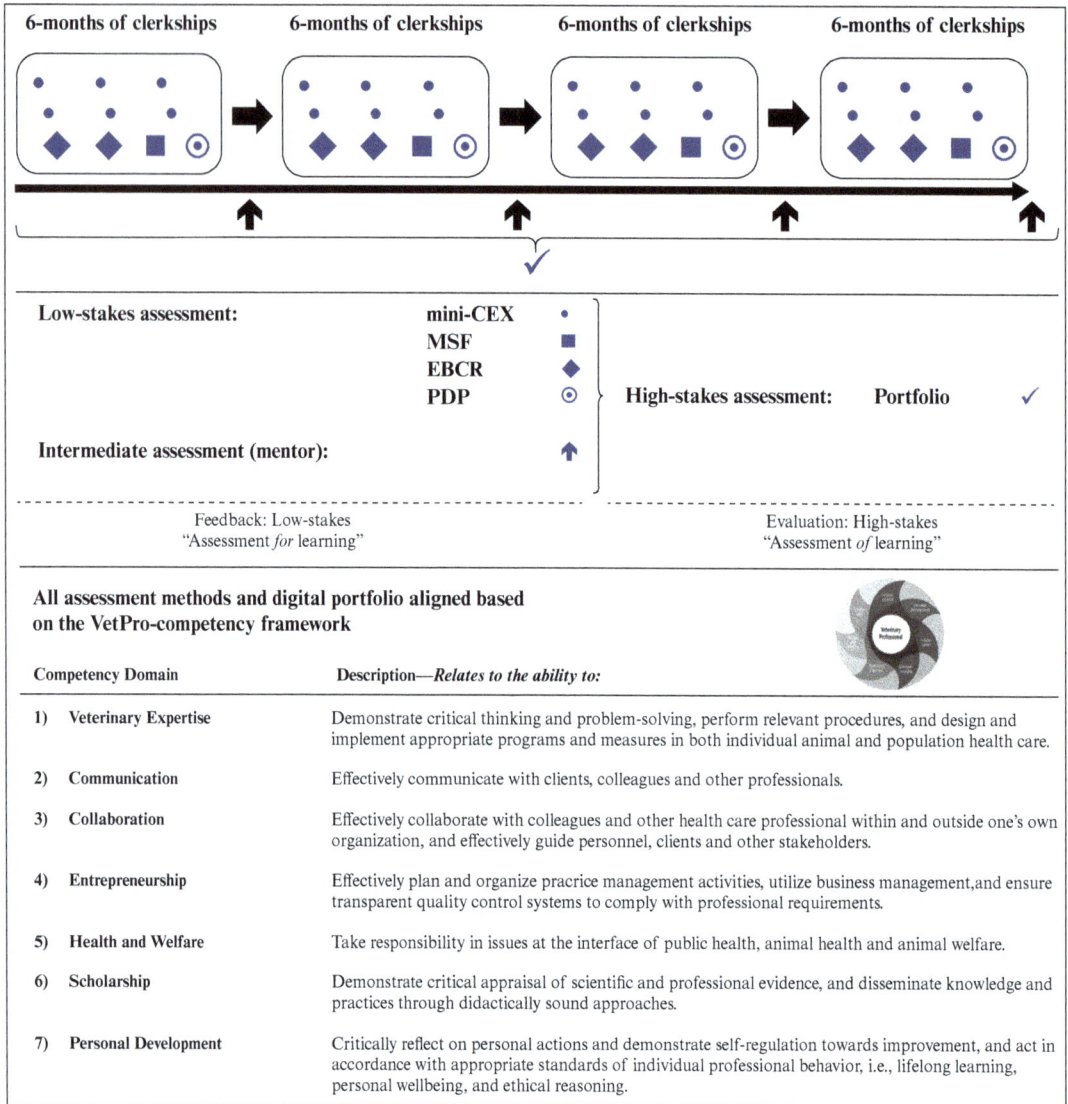

Figure 6-4 • Schematic overview of competency-based assessment program at the Faculty of Veterinary Medicine, Utrecht University. mini-CEX; MSF—multisource feedback; EBCR—evidence-based case report; PDP—personal development plan. Reproduced with permission from Bok et al. 2018 [51].

assurance process. Regular evaluations take place, including internal evaluations of each clinical rotation as well as a final evaluation of the entire clinical program at graduation. Furthermore, student representatives are members of all educational committees responsible for safeguarding the quality of the educational program, thereby representing their peers' voice. Finally, scientific research is part of the quality assurance processes. There is also a research group specifically devoted to improving quality in veterinary education, including research on validity evidence within programmatic assessment. Over the years, this has resulted in a vast amount of scientific publications that directly serve as input for quality assurance measures.

Various strategies are implemented to foster the trustworthiness of the high-stakes decision. Herein the FVMU applied the same framework derived from literature as the PCI program (previous case) [8]. Even though both program strategies are the same, the examples illustrate that the approach differs in practice. For a detailed overview, see Table 6-4 [8]. FVMU's competency committee consists of approximately 11 members who have have different roles within the program (e.g., clinician, teacher, scientists). All members are trained before performing high-stakes decision-making. The training includes instructions on the use of the e-portfolio system and side-by-side training in performing high-stakes decisions by one or more committee members. An important selection criterion for competency committee members is their acquaintance with the assessment program (i.e., being involved as a WBA tool assessor or otherwise having demonstrable knowledge of the program). To prevent potential conflicts of interest of the assessor, the assessors are asked to point out if they feel there could be a potential conflict of interest (e.g., extensively worked with the students, student–mentor relationship). If so, student affairs assign a different assessor to that portfolio.

To ensure that the decision-making process is auditable (transparent and defensible), the processes involved in high-stakes decision-making are documented and shared with the student. An assessment form is applied in which each competency domain is described on milestone levels accompanied with a narrative explanation. At the end of the form the assessor provides the student with overall feedback on the student's strengths and weaknesses. Previous research has shown a high percentage of agreement between the two independent assessors [52].

Another important aspect of a defensible decision is the provision of sufficient information about the students' performance. The high-stakes decisions of the portfolio are based on a multitude of data points, including multiple assessment methods, varying assessors, and contexts. A big data study performed at the FVMU showed that the milestone scores are reliable and capable of differentiating between students [51].

The program is reviewed externally by various accreditation bodies with a positive outcome: NVAO, the accreditation organization of the Netherlands and Flanders; AVMA, the American Veterinary Medical Association; CVMA, the Canadian Veterinary Medical Association; and

Table 6-4   QUALITATIVE RESEARCH STRATEGIES AND CRITERIA AND SOME EXAMPLES OF ASSESSMENT STRATEGIES FOR BUILDING TRUSTWORTHINESS IN ASSESSMENT DECISIONS

Strategies to Establish Trustworthiness	Criterion	Assessment Strategy	Examples of Strategies Used in the Program
Credibility	Prolonged engagement	• Training of assessors • The persons who know the student the best (mentor, peers) provide information for the assessment. • Incorporate intermittent feedback cycles in the procedure.	• Organizing workshops for clinical teachers and mentors • Development of informative e-module • Training students • Establish clear guidelines • Regular calibration sessions competency committee
	Triangulation	• Many assessors should be involved, and different credible groups should be included. • Use multiple sources of assessment within or across methods. • Organize a sequential judgment procedure in which conflicting information necessitates the gathering of more information.	• Use a variety of assessor groups (peers, clinical teachers, patient owners, etc.). • Applications of different assessment tools • Have mentor system (intermediate stake) and two independent assessors (high stake).
	Peer examination or peer debriefing	• Organize discussion between assessors (before and intermediate) for benchmarking and discussion of the process and the results. • Separate multiple roles of the assessors by removing the summative assessment decisions from the coaching role.	• Informal meetings of clinical teams • Independent competency committee

	Method	Strategy	Example
	Member checking	• Incorporate the learner's point of view in the assessment procedure. • Incorporate in the procedure intermittent feedback cycles.	• Include PDPs and reports of the student–mentor meetings • Organize frequent mentor meetings.
	Structural coherence	• Organize assessment committee to discuss inconsistencies in the assessment data.	• Mentor meetings and independent competency committee procedure
Transferability	Time sampling	• Sample broadly over different contexts and patients.	• Allow data to be collected over a prolonged period of time.
	Thick description (or dense description)	• Incorporate in the assessment instruments possibilities to give qualitative, narrative information. • Give narrative information a lot of weight in the assessment procedure.	• WBA tools, notes, PDP forms and reports of student–mentor meetings • Milestones • Train competency committee members
Dependability	Stepwise replication	• Broad sampling over different assessors	• Assessment activities over different clinical rotations
Dependability or confirmability	Audit	• Document the different steps in the assessment process (a formal assessment plan approved by an examination committee, overviews of the results per phase). • Organize quality assessment procedures with external auditor. • Give learners the possibility to appeal to the assessment decision.	• e-portfolio • Have supportive documents and an e-module provide a clear outline of the requirements • Several audits have been performed. • There is a clearly documented appeals procedure.

EAEVE, the European Association of Establishments for Veterinary Education.

Lessons Learned

The main lesson we learned is the importance of the implementation process. This includes the involvement of different stakeholders, with specific attention to the involvement of students. Herein communication plays a significant role in keeping all stakeholders up to date on the developments and choices made and to give them the opportunity to voice their thoughts during the implementation process. This communication does not stop after implementation; continuously updating all stakeholders is important. Another crucial aspect is changing the assessment culture. There has always been a profound notion of the importance of summative testing and providing grades; this is incredibly difficult, and patience is key. Also, aspects like faculty development and allocating time for observation and feedback in daily clinical practice are beneficial strategies in transforming the assessment culture. In implementing a programmatic approach, there is a refocus on assessment for learning. To achieve this, there should be a sustainable feedback culture [53,54].

▌ IMPLICATIONS FOR QUALITY ASSURANCE

In programmatic assessment, the main focus is on the program as an entity instead of one single assessment method. This requires viewing assessment and quality assurance as a complex system, with multiple interconnected components and processes. In the literature, multiple frameworks for quality assurance have been proposed at the program level: for example, quality criteria for competence assessment programs by Baartman et al. [55], a practical tool to analyze the strengths and deficiencies in the program of assessment by Bierer et al. [29], a framework for systems of assessments by Norcini et al. [7], and the use of criteria originating from qualitative research quality indicators, and trustworthiness by van der Vleuten et al. [8]. These frameworks can be used as guides to evaluate quality assurance in programmatic assessment. For a more elaborated theoretical foundation of the processes involved in quality assurance on program level, please see **Chapter 9**.

In this section, the CCLCM, PCI, and FVMU case has been used to highlight themes these different contexts prioritized and addressed in their quality assurance processes. Through data presentation and deliberate

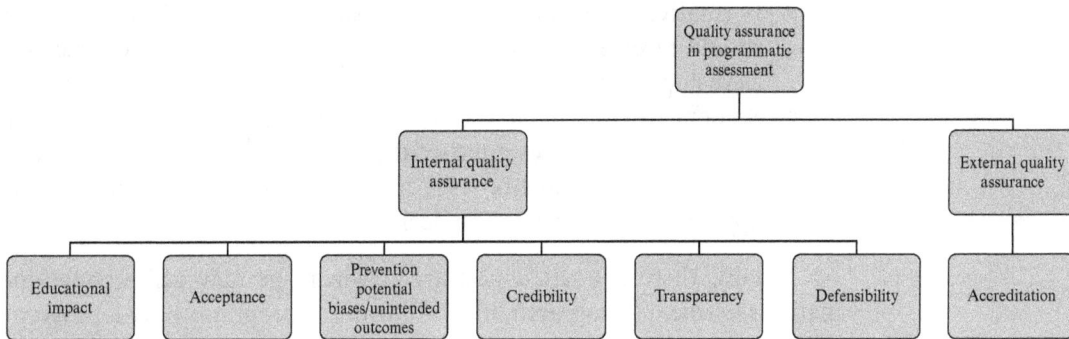

Figure 6-5 • Overview of the different themes present in quality assurance measures in programmatic assessment.

discussion, the authors (LJ, HB, BB, and CV) derived emerging themes within the quality assurance processes of the presented programs. Figure 6-5 shows an overview of these themes as a potential guide for designing quality assurance practices in a programmatic approach to assessment. Note that these themes are neither prescriptive nor exhaustive but should be seen as themes that could be considered in designing quality assurance processes in a programmatic approach to assessment.

External Quality Assurance
As already highlighted in **Chapters 1** and **2**, quality assurance comprises both internal and external quality assurance. External quality assurance includes external audits and accreditation. Accreditation is crucial in guaranteeing that the program meets certain national or international standards. Accreditation standards focus strongly on whether programs achieve the desired outcomes with their graduates. In a programmatic assessment system, this is relatively easy to demonstrate. For instance, the Liaison Committee on Medical Education (LCME) is the accreditation body for all MD degree programs in the United States and Canada [56]. The LCME has 12 standards with multiple subcomponents to inform accreditation decisions. Several LCME standards apply to programmatic assessment practices, as illustrated in the following list:

- Self-directed and Life-long Learning (Standard 6.3)—Students should have opportunities to self-assess their performance.
- Narrative Assessment (Standard 9.5)—Students should receive narrative written feedback about their performance during every course and clerkship.

- Formative Assessment and Feedback (Standard 9.7)—Students should receive feedback in sufficient time during every course and clerkship to remediate performance.
- Student Advancement and Appeal Processes (Standard 9.9)—Fair and formal processes must exist for progression decisions, including providing students with the opportunity to respond to or appeal adverse progression decisions.

Finally, there is a discussion about when one may call a programmatic assessment "programmatic." All training programs have a program of assessment, but that is not the same as programmatic assessment. A program is truly programmatic when it adheres to the building blocks described previously in this chapter. These building blocks can be implemented in many different ways, and programmatic assessment programs may have many different manifestations.

Internal Quality Assurance

Educational impact

A unique feature in programmatic assessment is the integration of (1) assessment *for* learning and (2) assessment *of* learning. However, the educational impact of the assessment program (assessment *for* learning) can easily be overlooked when embracing quality assurance measures. In our opinion, evaluating the educational impact is imperative in a well-functioning assessment system, including:

- Provision of high-quality and meaningful feedback to the learner (at the CCLCM, for example, the PBL facilitators receive training in providing rich narratives),
- Monitoring the extent to which students and faculty perceive the learning environment as positive; and
- Fostering students' reflective practice abilities (ensuring a rigorous mentoring system that includes a pool of qualified and accessible mentors is highly recommended).

Acceptance

The assessment program and its procedures should be accepted by all stakeholders. For example, students should understand the assessment procedure and its relevance. To facilitate this, comprehension of the assessment program by all stakeholders (assessment literacy) is important—for example, by training and writing clear documents about portfolio requirements. Also, adequate resources should be provided to faculty to perform assessments. At the CCLCM, for example, longitudinal clinical preceptors have shortened clinical schedules during days when supervising students in ambulatory clinics to allow them time to observe students directly and provide detailed narrative feedback. Acceptance is an important theme to address in programmatic assessment because the presented cases in this chapter illustrate that a successful implementation requires all stakeholders to be active agents in the process.

Prevention of Potential Biases and Unintended Outcomes

As with all assessments, there are potential biases and unintended outcomes. One major pitfall in a programmatic approach to assessment is when mentors, who are appointed to guide the learning process of the student, are involved in high-stakes decision-making. This is not desirable because learning should be separated from the high-stakes decision. The mentor could, however, provide valuable information to the competency committee. After all, he or she has seen the student frequently. At the PCI program, for example, the mentor provides a recommendation to the committee. Even if the mentoring system and the high-stakes decision are separated, members of the competency committee are often involved in teaching or coaching practices. This might result in potential conflicts of interest. For example, the student is a mentee of the committee member or the committee member has had a previous negative encounter with the student. Furthermore, there could potentially be unintended outcomes that are more difficult to forecast. To prevent these, the program could monitor if there are indications of potential unintended outcomes. For example, at the CCLCM, evaluations take place on whether the assessment system places students at a disadvantage when applying for residency programs.

Credibility

The assessment program should be perceived as being credible by all stakeholders. Faculty development is a major component of ensuring credibility. To establish high-quality faculty development, a well-thought system should be designed focusing on faculty involved in (1) coaching practices, (2) high-stakes decision-making, and (3) WBAs. Practices include training in coaching or provision of meaningful feedback and regular meetings to share best practices. Furthermore, credibility can be established by the design of the assessment procedure. For example, the high-stakes decision is made in groups (competency committee) or the intermediate assessment by another mentor (PCI program).

Transparency

The assessment procedure should be transparent to all stakeholders and should be fair for all students. Various procedures can be built in to ensure transparency. These include (1) keeping an updated audit trail of the assessment process, including all choices and considerations; (2) having a clear documentation of the assessment program; (3) providing an appeals procedure to the students; (4) having an examination committee appointed to regularly check the assessment procedure; and (5) monitoring the extent to which all students have equal or comparable learning experiences.

Defensibility

The high-stakes decision should be defensible. To fulfill this, there should be (1) sufficient assessment data, (2) a representative sample of low-stakes assessments, and (3) assessment instruments that align with the intended outcomes. Sufficient assessment data and a representative sample can be generated through a variety of methods, contexts, and assessors and by including multiple time points and having a profound focus on providing qualitative information. For example, the FVMU has documented requirements for the number of low-stakes data points to be included in the portfolio.

Continued Evaluation Process

As a final note, the process of quality assurance is preferably a continued process that involves different stakeholders, especially current and (former) students and assessment committee members who can potentially be important sources of information. Focus groups, questionnaires, informal feedback meetings, and one-on-one interviews are examples of methods to exert in this process. For instance, the CCLCM program conducts exit interviews with all graduates to obtain their perceptions of the assessment system and educational program and solicits feedback (questionnaire) from alumni following the first year of residency training and 10 years postgraduation. In addition to this, CCLCM seeks feedback from residency program directors about graduates' preparation for and performance during residency. Also, a continued evaluation can include conducting scientific research. At the PCI program, multiple research projects are gathering empirical evidence around programmatic assessment.

▌CONCLUSION

Because programmatic assessment embodies current developments within modern assessment strategies, it has increasingly been implemented worldwide. In this chapter, three cases adopting a programmatic approach to assessment were presented. These examples not only illustrate various reasons to change but also show that programmatic assessment can be successfully implemented within different contexts despite the hurdles to overcome. Furthermore, even though each implementation operationalized its own quality assurance processes, the authors address common themes concerning both internal and external processes. These themes are neither prescriptive nor exhaustive but should rather be seen as themes that could be considered when designing quality assurance processes in a programmatic approach to assessment.

▌REFERENCES

1. Cilliers FJ, Schuwirth LW, Herman N, Adendorff HJ, van der Vleuten CPM. A Model of the Pre-Assessment Learning Effects of Summative Assessment in Medical Education. *Adv Health Sci Educ*. 2012;17(1):39–53.
2. Shute VJ. Focus on Formative Feedback. *Rev Educ Res*. 2008;78(1):153–189.
3. Harrison CJ, Könings KD, Dannefer EF, et al. Factors Influencing Students' Receptivity to Formative Feedback Emerging from Different Assessment Cultures. *Perspect Med Educ*. 2016;5(5):276–284.
4. Van der Vleuten CPM, Schuwirth LW. Assessing Professional Competence: From Methods to Programmes. *Med Educ*. 2005;39(3):309–317.
5. Frank JR, Snell LS, ten Cate O, et al. Competency-Based Medical Education: Theory to Practice. *Med Teach*. 2010;32(8):638–645.
6. Carraccio C, Wolfsthal SD, Englander R, Ferentz K, Martin C. Shifting Paradigms: From Flexner to Competencies. *Acad Med*. 2002;77(5):361–367.
7. Norcini J, Anderson MB, Bollela V, et al. 2018 Consensus Framework for Good Assessment. *Med Teach*. 2018;40(11):1102–1109.
8. Van der Vleuten C, Schuwirth L, Scheele F, Driessen EW, Hodges B. The Assessment of Professional Competence: Building Blocks for Theory Development. *Best Pract Res Cl Ob*. 2010;24(6):703–719.
9. Van der Vleuten C, Schuwirth L, Driessen EW, et al. A Model for Programmatic Assessment Fit for Purpose. *Med Teach*. 2012;34(3):205–214.
10. Schuwirth LW, van der Vleuten CPM. Programmatic Assessment: From Assessment of Learning to Assessment for Learning. *Med Teach*. 2011;33(6): 478–485.
11. Bacon R, Kellett J, Dart J, et al. A Consensus Model: Shifting Assessment Practices in Dietetics Tertiary Education. *Nutr Diet*. 2018;75(4):418–430.
12. Dannefer EF, Henson LC. The Portfolio Approach to Competency-Based Assessment at the Cleveland Clinic Lerner College of Medicine. *Acad Med*. 2007;82(5):493–502.
13. Chan T, Sherbino J. The McMaster Modular Assessment Program (McMAP): A Theoretically Grounded Work-Based Assessment System for an Emergency Medicine Residency Program. *Acad Med*. 2015;90(7):900–905.
14. Rich JV, Fostaty Young S, Donnelly C, et al. Competency-Based Education Calls for Programmatic Assessment: But What Does This Look Like in Practice? *J Eval Clin Pract*. 2020;26(4):1087–1095.

15. Lurie SJ, Mooney CJ, Lyness JM. Measurement of the General Competencies of the Accreditation Council for Graduate Medical Education: A Systematic Review. *Acad Med.* 2009;84(3):301–309.

16. Swing SR. The ACGME Outcome Project: Retrospective and Prospective. *Med Teach.* 2007;29(7):648–654.

17. Fishleder AJ, Henson LC, Hull AL. Cleveland Clinic Lerner College of Medicine: An Innovative Approach to Medical Education and the Training of Physician Investigators. *Acad Med.* 2007;82(4):390–396.

18. Wyngaarden JB. The Clinical Investigator as an Endangered Species. *N Engl J Med.* 1979;301(23):1254–1259.

19. Milewicz DM, Lorenz RG, Dermody TS, Brass LF. Rescuing the Physician-Scientist Workforce: The Time for Action Is Now. *J Clin Invest.* 2015;125(10): 3742–3747.

20. Rosenberg LE. The Physician-Scientist: An Essential—and Fragile—Link in the Medical Research Chain. *J Clin Invest.* 1999;103(12):1621–1626.

21. Zemlo TR, Garrison HH, Partridge NC, Ley TJ. The Physician-Scientist: Career Issues and Challenges at the Year 2000. *FASEB J.* 2000;14(2):221–230.

22. Dannefer EF. Beyond Assessment of Learning Toward Assessment for Learning: Educating Tomorrow's Physicians. *Med Teach.* 2013;35(7):560–563.

23. Dijkstra J, van der Vleuten CPM, Schuwirth LWT. A New Framework for Designing Programmes of Assessment. *Adv Health Sci Educ.* 2010;15(3):379–393.

24. Dannefer EF, Bierer SB, Gladding SP. Evidence Within a Portfolio-Based Assessment Program: What Do Medical Students Select to Document Their Performance? *Med Teach.* 2012;34(3):215–220.

25. Bierer SB, Dannefer EF, Taylor C, Hall P, Hull AL. Methods to Assess Students' Acquisition, Application and Integration of Basic Science Knowledge in an Innovative Competency-Based Curriculum. *Med Teach.* 2008;30(7):e171–e177.

26. Altahawi F, Sisk B, Poloskey S, Hicks C, Dannefer EF. Student Perspectives on Assessment: Experience in a Competency-Based Portfolio System. *Med Teach.* 2012;34(3):221–225.

27. Bierer SB, Dannefer EF. The Learning Environment Counts: Longitudinal Qualitative Analysis of Study Strategies Adopted by First-Year Medical Students in a Competency-Based Educational Program. *Acad Med.* 2016;91(11):S44–S52.

28. Bierer SB, Dannefer EF, Tetzlaff JE. Time to Loosen the Apron Strings: Cohort-Based Evaluation of a Learner-Driven Remediation Model at One Medical School. *J Gen Intern Med.* 2015;30(9):1339–1343.

29. Bierer SB, Colbert CY, Foshee CM, French JC, Pien LC. Tool for Diagnosing Gaps within a Competency-Based Assessment System. *Acad Med.* 2018;93(3):512.

30. Frank JR, Danoff D. The CanMEDS Initiative: Implementing an Outcomes-Based Framework of Physician Competencies. *Med Teach.* 2007;29(7):642–647.

31. Diemers AD, van de Wiel MWJ, Scherpbier AJ, Heineman E, Dolmans DH. Pre-Clinical Patient Contacts and the Application of Biomedical and Clinical Knowledge. *Med Educ.* 2011;45(3):280–288.

32. Van der Vleuten CP, Schuwirth LW. Assessment in the Context of Problem-Based Learning. *Adv Health Sci Educ.* 2019;24(5):903–914.

33. Wrigley W, van der Vleuten CPM, Freeman A, Muijtjens A. A Systemic Framework for the Progress Test: Strengths, Constraints and Issues—AMEE Guide No. 71. *Med Teach*. 2012;34(9):683–697.

34. Ravesloot CJ, van der Schaaf MF, Muijtjens A, et al. The Don't Know Option in Progress Testing. *Adv Health Sci Educ*. 2015;20(5):1325–1338.

35. Van der Vleuten C, Schuwirth L, Muijtjens A, et al. Cross Institutional Collaboration in Assessment: A Case on Progress Testing. *Med Teach*. 2004;26(8):719–725.

36. Collares CF, Cecilio-Fernandes D. When I Say… Computerised Adaptive Testing. *Med Educ*. 2019;53(2):115–116.

37. Van der Vleuten C, Freeman A, Collares CF. Progress Test Utopia. *Perspect Med Educ*. 2018;7(2):136–138.

38. Van Mook WN, de Grave WS, Wass V, et al. Professionalism: Evolution of the Concept. *Eur J Intern Med*. 2009;20(4):e81–e84.

39. Van Luijk SJ, Smeets JGE, Smits J, Wolfhagen I, Perquin MLF. Assessing Professional Behaviour and the Role of Academic Advice at the Maastricht Medical School. *Med Teach*. 2000;22(2):168–172.

40. Dolmans DHJM, Wolfhagen HAP, Scherpbier AJJA. From Quality Assurance to Total Quality Management: How Can Quality Assurance Result in Continuous Improvement in Health Professions Education? *Educ Health*. 2003;16(2):210–217.

41. Frambach JM, van der Vleuten CPM, Durning SJ. AM Last Page: Quality Criteria in Qualitative and Quantitative Research. *Acad Med*. 2013;88(4):552.

42. Schut S, Driessen E, van Tartwijk J, van der Vleuten C, Heeneman S. Stakes in the Eye of the Beholder: An International Study of Learners' Perceptions within Programmatic Assessment. *Med Educ*. 2018;52(6):654–663.

43. Schut S, van Tartwijk J, Driessen E, van der Vleuten C, Heeneman S. Understanding the Influence of Teacher–Learner Relationships on Learners' Assessment Perception. *Adv Health Sci Educ*. 2020;25(2):441–456.

44. Heeneman S, de Grave W. Tensions in Mentoring Medical Students Toward Self-Directed and Reflective Learning in a Longitudinal Portfolio-Based Mentoring System—An Activity Theory Analysis. *Med Teach*. 2017;39(4):368–376.

45. Heeneman S, Schut S, Donkers J, van der Vleuten C, Muijtjens A. Embedding of the Progress Test in an Assessment Program Designed According to the Principles of Programmatic Assessment. *Med Teach*. 2017;39(1):44–52.

46. Van der Vleuten CP. Revisiting 'Assessing Professional Competence: From Methods to Programmes'. *Med Educ*. 2016;50(9):885–888.

47. Collins A, Joseph D, Bielaczyc K. Design Research: Theoretical and Methodological Issues. *The J Learn Sci*. 2004;13(1):15–42.

48. Bok HG, Jaarsma DA, Teunissen PW, van der Vleuten CPM, van Beukelen P. Development and Validation of a Competency Framework for Veterinarians. *J Vet Med Educ*. 2011;38(3):262–269.

49. Korthagen FA, Kessels J, Koster B, Lagerwerf B, Wubbels T. *Linking Practice and Theory: The Pedagogy of Realistic Teacher Education*. Routledge; 2001.

50. Ten Cate TJ, ter Braak E, Frenkel J, van de Pol AC. De 4-tot-10 verwacht niveauschaal (410VN-schaal) bij persoonlijke beoordelingen. *Tijdschrift voor Medisch Onderwijs*. 2006;25(4):157–163.

51. Bok HG, de Jong LH, O'Neill T, Maxey C, Hecker KG. Validity Evidence for Programmatic Assessment in Competency-Based Education. *Perspect Med Educ*. 2018;7(6):362–372.

52. De Jong LH, Bok HG, Kremer WD, van der Vleuten CPM. Programmatic Assessment: Can We Provide Evidence for Saturation Of Information? *Med Teach*. 2019;41(6):678–682.

53. Bok HG, Teunissen PW, Spruijt A, et al. Clarifying Students' Feedback-Seeking Behaviour in Clinical Clerkships. *Med Educ*. 2013;47(3):282–291.

54. De Jong LH, Favier RP, van der Vleuten CPM, Bok HG. Students' Motivation Toward Feedback-Seeking in the Clinical Workplace. *Med Teach*. 2017;39(9):954–958.

55. Baartman LK, Bastiaens TJ, Kirschner PA, van der Vleuten CPM. The Wheel of Competency Assessment: Presenting Quality Criteria for Competency Assessment Programs. *Stud Educ Evaluation*. 2006;32(2):153–170.

56. Liaison Committee on Medical Education. Functions and Structures of a Medical School. 2020. Retrieved from https://lcme.org/publications/#Standards.

The Role of Technology in the Quality Assurance of Assessment Processes

7

Filipe Falcão, Patrício Costa, and José Miguel Pêgo

CHAPTER HIGHLIGHTS

- Technology is changing the landscape of assessment in medical education.
- Computer-based testing increases efficiency and flexibility of assessment.
- Machine learning adds realism and reliability to assessment.

ORIENTATION TO THE CHAPTER

In this chapter, we will address the impact of the latest technological developments in quality processes regarding assessment in medical education.

In the first part, we discuss the evolution of assessment in medical education and how the growing need for assessment opportunities has nudged traditional formats toward computer-based assessment. In the second part, we look at how technology is impacting foundational tasks in assessment in particular, test design, test assembly, and reporting. In the third part, we will analyze how technology is impacting operationally and improving efficiency and accuracy of assessments. Finally, we will elaborate on what we envision the future holds for assessment in medical education.

INTRODUCTION—THE INCREASING ROLE OF TECHNOLOGY IN MEDICINE AND MEDICAL EDUCATION

Profound global and economic changes are changing educational measurement [1]. Thanks to the unified effort of cognitive sciences, statistical theories of test scores, education psychology, educational technology, and computer science, educational measurement is evolving at a fast pace. This exponential evolution translates into clear changes in the assessment systems, the most notable of which is the transition from assessment through paper tests to computer tests [2]. This change reveals a shift in the paradigm of educational assessment, with paper-based tests being no longer a feasible method because of its resource-intensive process, which urged for solutions like computer-based testing (CBT) systems [3,4,5]. In fact, over the last few years, CBT has become a widely used form of evaluation and is now considered one of the most effective assessment methodologies in education [6].

Computer-Based Testing

CBT is changing educational measurement due to the merging of test-administration procedures with digital media and the Internet, which makes it possible to create new types of tests and testing resources. These tests are paperless and administered with a computer that uses a test model to implement a process of selecting and administering items, allowing the students' performances to be scored and categorized by their ability in each item [2]. According to the authors, this approach has potential benefits such as shortened tests without loss of measurement precision; enhanced score reliability, particularly for low- and high-ability examinees; improved test security; testing on demand; and immediate test scoring and reporting.

The introduction of the Internet and the proliferation of Internet-based computerized assessment has further improved this scoring system, making it especially advantageous for both educators and students when compared with traditional testing methods [2,7]. Through the administration of tests over the network, educators not only are free of time-consuming processes usually associated with paper-based tests but also are able to use more diverse item formats that can measure a broader range of skills. Students also profit from this approach, sometimes being able to take exams when and where they want, as well as receive immediate feedback on their performance thanks to computerized algorithms that allow the immediate quotation of their tests [5,8].

Medical education stands out as one of the areas where this change in assessment methodologies has become evident, introducing new teaching and learning strategies that allow medical educators to measure complex performances and competencies [9,10]. Consequently, medical examinations once administered in paper format are now delivered through computers connected to the Internet. Computers allow the use of item types that help medical educators measure performances and a broad set of competencies, as well as provide continuous on-demand testing and instantaneous feedback [10].

Measurement in medical education environment is an extremely complex task because it involves a variety of competences and settings [11]. Medical educators are constantly challenged with teaching demands that reflect the continuous growth in scientific information and society's expectations of the universe of knowledge that medical doctors must master to be fit for the profession [11]. Consequently, there is a constant conflict between education and research related to funding, time, and promotional aspects [11]. Because of this expectation and the inadequacies of training models, medical education experienced great pressure to transform, which took medical educators to seek better evaluation tools like CBT [12]. This search for assessment tools that support learning and measure performance is also a reaction against old methods of assessment that had adverse effect on both learners and teachers, which culminated in new assessment strategies to meet these needs of innovation [9] and quality improvement [9,11].

Assessment in medical education has three main goals: (1) optimize the capabilities of learners, directing them to future learning; (2) protect the public through the identification of doctors not fit for the job; and (3) provide a platform for choosing applicants for complex training [11]. According to these authors, assessment in this area can be classified into one of two types: (1) *formative*, which provides guidance for future learning, promotes reflections and reassurance, and shapes values; and (2) *summative*, which consists of an overall judgment regarding the competence or qualification of the learner.

According to the same authors [11], one of the main evaluation methodologies in this area is the written exam with open-ended or Multiple Choice Questions (MCQs). The latter are the foundation for assessments used in medical education [13] because of their capacity to provide broad sampling of knowledge in many areas and domains of specialization, using larger sets of items, which makes other methodologies impractical [13,14]. In addition, they can be scored by computers, which can help administer them in an even shorter period [11]. They are also particularly advantageous for evaluating medical students due to their ability of testing a large number of candidates with reduced human intervention being efficient and economic [13,15]. In the medical context, MCQs measure the breadth and ability of graduate and postgraduate students within a particular specialty, standing out for their objectivity, efficiency, increased quantity, and item statistics that help discern their psychometric qualities [14].

However, CBT brought new challenges, particularly in item development [2,16]. In fact, the growth of Internet-based computerized testing warned of the needs for new testing methods and practices [7]. Since these tests are continually applied and consequently exposed, thousands of items are necessary to develop item banks—pools of test items containing information regarding their content and psychometric details such as difficulty—that need to be constantly replenished to minimize these risks [1,10]. In medical education, in addition to the demands of larger item banks, there are problems related to the implementation of MCQs such as the time and money spent on their construction [10,14]. Although the creation of MCQ follows guidelines that allow the development of items across different specializations, this process is complex because cognitive problem-solving skills and content knowledge should be expressed by specialists and replicated countless times [13]. These items are also not free of validity problems, which calls for more alternative methods of test development [10,15].

As a result of this transition to computerized testing, the demand for new items is now greater than the supply in educational assessment [3,17]. Educational items as they are currently produced are expensive and time-consuming [1]. In the traditional method, developers are hired to extend the traditional approach of content experts, which consists in creating one item at a time [16]. This approach to the development of content items requires "experts to use test specifications, and item-writing guides to author each item" [2], which is an expensive process because of the need to hire experts.

Although feasible for classroom assessments, this method is difficult to apply in large-scale examinations [13]. Extensive MCQ development is necessary to create items needed for medical licensure examinations [13]. In addition to the costs of hiring specialists, there are costs related to item quality control, which implies that all items must be field-tested before their use to measure their psychometric characteristics (sometimes resulting in the elimination of a large number of items). Because educators now need to create a large number of new items for computerized testing, this process of writing, revision, and editing shows us that this traditional approach does not seem to be the most promising way to deal with this problem [1].

Automated Item Generation

Automated item generation (AIG) is a next-generation assessment theory that promises to overcome the challenges imposed by traditional item development and to smooth the item development burden for medical examinations [8,13,18]. AIG is an item construction technology in applied psychometrics that has attracted interest because of its potential capacity to produce high-quality and content-specific test items rapidly and efficiently [3,18]. It regards an area where computer technology, cognitive theories, and psychometric practices gather to conduct a process that can produce assessment tasks [1]. More specifically, it consists in the "process of using cognitive models to generate items using computer technology," thus providing a way to systematically produce a large number of items focused on a specific content both quickly and efficiently ([5], p. 6). Guided by psychometric theory of test items and aided by computer algorithms [20], it requires human judgment and expertise to define the elements in the item model and computers to combine these elements [13,14,20]. This requires content specialists to design and develop meaningful item models. Subsequently, computer technology systematically combines the elements of these item models to produce large numbers of test items, allowing the measurement of medical students' knowledge and problem-solving skills in different areas of medical education [2,13,20].

HOW TECHNOLOGY IS IMPACTING FOUNDATIONAL TASKS IN ASSESSMENT

Test Design

Test design includes all steps from the development of a blueprint, item development, test assembly, and test administration. In addition, postadministration tasks such as scoring and feedback provision depend on the purpose of the assessment but need to be thought about beforehand to understand its impact on the design of the test. All of these steps can be technologically enhanced, improving efficiency and the quality of the final design in some cases.

Item Development

As indicated in **Chapter 3**, item development is traditionally accomplished by an individual or group of content experts. College-sized institutions typically develop their assessments in-house, resorting to individual faculty members and groups in some cases. Less frequently are people specially dedicated to item development. On the other hand, licensing institutions such as certification boards and standard test developers frequently group content experts to develop a small number of high-quality items. Although in the first case, items usually tend to be of low cost and poor quality [21], certification-level items that are used in high-stakes examinations are expensive due to the extensive quality-control process [22].

The widespread use of computer-based assessment has helped ease this process by enforcing item templates and guiding authors toward the best item shape and format. In addition, CBTs provide item formats that are difficult or impossible to reproduce on paper such as multistep MCQs, hotspot, long-list items requiring video or audio recordings, and so on.

Recent developments have brought new avenues to item development and the final quality of the assessment that depends on computer technology such as automation of item development and the use of natural language processing and machine learning.

Automated Item Generation

To clearly understand the process of creating items through AIG, it is necessary to define some concepts—namely, item model, element, stem, option, and auxiliary information. According to Gierl and Lai [1], an item model is like a template that indicates the variables (elements) in the task that can be manipulated to create new items. More specifically, it is a general representation of the item to be generated, incorporating necessary properties of the items like the stem, options, and auxiliary information [23]. Gierl and Lai [1] claim that the stem is the part of the item model that contains the "context, content, [or] the question the student is required to answer" (p. 11)—that is, formulating the problem that the item addresses [23]. The options correspond to the possible answers to the item, where one is correct and one or more are incorrect. Finally, auxiliary information corresponds to support information regarding the item (e.g., image or tables) [1]. Further, the stem and options are divided into elements, which can be non-numeric or numeric (integers). Regarding MCQ item models, the stem and options are always required, whereas only the stem is necessary in open-ended response item models [7].

AIG usually requires two major steps. In the first, an item model is created derived from good-quality test items [23]. More specifically, a content specialist creates item models which elements in the task should be manipulated [1]. In the second step, these variables in the item model are varied through computer algorithms to generate new items. Once the item model is created by the content specialists, computer technology combines the elements specified by them in each model, producing a series of new items [1,23] called *isomorphs*—that is, clone items. With this two-step process, AIG can creates a large quantity of new items from one item model, ensuring that there are enough items for the item banks, which reflects the full potential of this technique in the future of assessment [1,18].

Regarding the generation of medical multiple choice items using AIG, Gierl et al. [13] list three steps. Unlike the process used in most item-generation techniques generated by AIG, the first step in medical evaluation is to create a cognitive model structure. (See Figure 7-1.) Here the content included in medical examinations is identified by the

COGNITIVE MODEL

PATIENT INFORMATION

DEMOGRAPHICS

Age
25 - 100
Constraints: > 65 Check Indications

Gender
Male, Female

If female (<45 yeras)

BLOOD PRESSURE

Category	Systolic	Diastolic
High-Normal	130-139	95-89
Grade 1	140-159	90-99
Grade 2	160-179	100-109
Grade 3	≥180	≥110

Pregnancy
Yes or No
Constraints: Check contraindications

RISK FACTORS

Personal or Family history of HT or Cardiovascular Disease
Personal or Family history of dyslipidemia
Personal History of Diabetes Mellitus
Smoking Habits
Obesity
Sleep Apnea

TREATMENT CONSTRAINTS

Gout
Asthma
AV Block
Peripheral Arterial Disease
Chronic Pulmonary Disease
Heart failure
Tachycardia
Angioedema
Hyperkalemia
Bilateral Renal Artery Stenosis
Kidney failure

TREATMENT CONDITIONS

CV RISCK

Blood Pressure / Risk Factors	High Normal SBP 130-139 or DBP 85-89	Grade 1 HT SBP 140-159 or DBP 90-99	Grade 2 HT SBP 160-179 or DBP 100-109	Grade 3 HT SBP > 180 or DBP > 110
No other risk factors	Average risk	Low added risk	Moderate added risk	High added risk
1-2 risk factors	Low added risk	Moderate added risk	Moderate added risk	Very High added risk
3 risk factors or Diabetes	High added risk	High added risk	High added risk	Very High added risk

DRUG CONTRAINDICATIONS

	Compelling	Possible
Thiazide diuretics	Gout	Metabolic syndrome Glucose intolerance Pregnancy
Beta Blockers	Asthma A-V block (grade 2/3)	Peripheral artery disese Glucose intolerance Athletes and physically active patients
Calcium Antagonists	A-V block (grade 2/3) Heart failure	Tachyarrhythmias
ACE inhibitors	Pregnancy Angioneurotic oedema Hyperkalaemia Bilateral renal artery stenosis	
ARA	Pregnancy Hyperkalaemia Bilateral renal artery stenosis	

SPECIFIC DRUG INDICATION

Renal failure	ACEi, ARB
Diabetes Mellitus	ACEi, ARB
Isolated systolic hypertension (elderly >65y)	Thiazide diuretics

TREATMENT

Initial Treatment

High-Normal or Grade 1, Low or Moderate added risk

Grade 2 or Grade 3, High or Very High added risk

Monotherapy Treatment
Thiazide diuretics
Beta Blockers
Calcium Antagonists
ACE inhibitors
ARB
Loop diuretics
Potassium-sparing diuretic

Combination of 2 drug treatment
Recommended combinations:
Thiazide + ACEi
ACEi + Calcium Antagonists
Thiazide + ARB
ARB + Calcium Antagonists
Thiazide + Calcium Antagonists
Beta Blockers + Calcium Antagonists

ITEM MODEL

QUESTION LABEL

[gender], [age] years, [if pregnant], presents [systolic blood pressure]/[Diastolic blood pressure]

This patient also as history of [Risk factors].

POSSIBLE QUESTIONS

Which hypertension grade does this patient fit in?

What is the Cardiovascular risk of this patient?

Which of these drugs class is contraindicated/indicated for this patient?

What is the most indicated drug (s) in this case?

The patient returns to the clinic after 6 months with a diagnosis of [New factor conditioning treatment]? Which of these classes of drug can not be prescribed, now?

Figure 7-1 • Top: Example of a cognitive model and respective item model. Bottom: Two examples of items derived from the cognitive model.

A 43-year-old man comes to the medical office. The patient has a history of tachyarrhythmia. Physical examination shows blood pressure of 131/87 mm Hg. What is the absolute risk of this patient?

A. Average risk
B. Low added risk
C. Average added risk
D. High added risk

A 52-year-old man comes to the medical office. The patient has a history of home measured morning blood pressure of 145/95 mm Hg. What degree of hypertension does this patient have?

A. Isolated systolic hypertension
B. Grade 1 hypertension
C. Grade 2 hypertension
D. Grade 3 hypertension

specialists, who outline a framework that structures the knowledge, skills, and content necessary to create a medical diagnosis, forming a cognitive model structure for AIG—that is, the experts summarize how they usually approach a problem [22]. This model organizes cognitive and content-specific information, presenting the content relationships and sources of information used to formulate medical diagnoses ([13], p.47). The second step consists in the development of the item models. More specifically, in this step the content of the cognitive model structure is cast to an MCQ, including the necessary information to generate a group of items. Variables to be altered are specified, vignettes including the information needed to answer a question are written, questions and correct options are defined, and distractors are generated [22,24]. Finally, the third step corresponds to the generation of items using item models through computer algorithms. Taking this process into account, we can consider AIG as a process by which the representation of students' thinking processes (cognitive models) are used to generate items thanks to computer algorithms [25].

Through the manipulation of the elements, specialists can generate a high number of items from just one item model, which can consequently modify the difficulty of an item. If the generated items were created with the objective of measuring contents at the same levels of difficulty, we consider the items to be isomorphic. In this case, only the incidental elements (or surface features of an item) are manipulated. On the other hand, when the goal is to create items with different difficulties, the incidental elements of the item model can be manipulated together with one or more radical elements (features that change item difficulty and test characteristics) [7].

However, AIG is not a rule-free process. It must follow standards of quality and guidelines for item-development practices that are initially used to identify a parent item model [13]. A *parent item model* refers to a high-quality item that "produce[s] strong item analysis results drawn from existing operation tests" (20, p. 46). A possible approach to identify a parent item model is through a cognitive theory of task performance. This approach is called *strong theory*, in which cognitive features are identified to control and predict test performance, which can help predict the difficulty of the generated items and, consequently, calibrate them without extensive pilot testing. However, these theories are rare. When a theory is not available, parent item models are identified through *weak theory*. In this approach, older items from other exams are reviewed "drawing on an inventory of existing test items" to identify an underlying structure that provides a reference to create alternative item models with features that can be changed to generate new items ([7], p. 278).

Another important point to consider is the taxonomy of the created item models. Item models can be (1) independent, (2) dependent, (3) mixed, or (4) fixed. This classification depends on the elements of the stem and the options of the model. In independent item models, the elements of the stem are unrelated, and a change in one element will not affect other elements. On the other hand, in dependent item models, those elements are causally related, whereas in mixed independent or dependent models at least one pair of the elements of the stem are related. Finally, fixed-item models are models where the stem elements have no variation. Regarding the options, they may be fixed (when distracters—plausible but incorrect alternatives [25]—and the right option are invariant in the item model), presented randomly, or in a constrained way (distracters are generated according to constraints). After the process of item model development and taxonomy is defined properly, AIG is ready to start. Through the aid of computer algorithms, item models are used to generate items and item banks [7].

The use of algorithms to generate items in education has the appeal that it may be able to produce unlimited resources for assessment development [26]. In addition to being a scalable process because it creates a large volume of items [3], AIG promises also to increase exam security through large sets of items with equal levels of difficulty [27], helping test developers identify tests that contains too many easy or difficult items. AIG can ease the development burden from the reuse of the item models instead of writing new items from scratch, avoiding errors that occur frequently during this phase (e.g., grammatical, punctuation, etc.) [3]. Because of these properties, we believe AIG can be used in medical schools, especially because their own item banks often have reduced numbers of items in certain areas of study [14].

Very Short Answer Questions

A very short answer question (VSAQ) is a novel type of item that can only be administered in CBTs. It consists of a clinical vignette followed by a question (usually about diagnosis or management) that requires a candidate to generate a short response [28]. The computer records these free-text answers (usually between one and four words) in a list of unique answers that can then be processed in a semiautomated way. Item developers can prepopulate the scoring system with a list of possible correct choices, and the assessment software can select correct answers by natural language processing. The advantage over traditional MCQs is that the cueing effect is absent, which has been shown to be an exceptionally reliable and discriminatory assessment method both in formative and summative examinations [28,29]. By eliminating cueing, it recreates real-life conditions of knowledge application and are candidates are better challenged. On the other hand, the list of answers that VSAQs collect can be used as distractors to develop classical MCQs. The advantage of this approach is that these are more likely to be better distractors and increase the discrimination power of classical MCQs because they represent the most common mistakes and misconceptions of test takers in a particular subject.

Test Form Assembly

Test form assembly is the process by which items in a particular assessment are arranged and presented to the test taker. This step is based on the blueprint of the test and can be extraordinarily complex, depending on the number of dimensions that have been defined for the blueprint. These dimensions are usually conditioned by the content (e.g., geometry, anatomy) being assessed by the item but may involve additional characteristics outside the content being sampled such as cognitive tasks being elicited (e.g., Bloom's taxonomy) and many more characteristics of the item that collectively constitute metadata associated with the item. Test assembly should be careful to ensure that the content is being comprehensively sampled without much overlap or underrepresentation of both content and metadata because these are important sources of information and feedback for both assessors and test takers. Computer-based assessment has changed how test form assembly is done, making it easier to classify items and manage item banks. Metadata can be easily associated with the item content and can be extraordinarily detailed. With specialized assessment software, it is possible to identify items associated to a particular characteristic and select them for the final test form. What was once a laborious process of manually picking items stored in text files and spreadsheets can be done with relative ease and automated to the point of fully autonomous assembly. Software can decide the specific set of items being included based on a blueprint of any dimensions but also taking into consideration the psychometric proprieties of items or the number of previous times used. This automation provides a randomly chosen sample of items that maximizes representation and avoids overlaps.

Another advantage of automated test assembly is the development of unique test forms for each test taker. Randomization of item order presentation is a method commonly used to avoid fraud and cheating. Paper-based test may include a few versions (usually three to five) of the same test form. Although it adds security, it also increases the workload needed to develop the test. Most software solutions, however, allow for the deployment of as many test forms as test takers, which reduces the risk of collusion and fraud. The level of randomization that computers can generate reduces the risk of assembling a test form that congregates too many difficult or easy items at the beginning or any other section of the form that has an emotional impact on test takers.

Scoring of Traditional and Novel Items

Test items traditionally fall into two categories: choice items and open answer (input items). Although open-answer items are highly flexible and allow for the evaluation of complex cognitive tasks such as synthetic ability, reasoning, and critical thinking, calculus, or design, they are more prone to bias in the scoring process. In addition, answering open-answer items may be labor and time intensive, which limits the number of items that can be included in one test form. The gain in freedom and realism provided by this category of item is counterbalanced by the limitation in sampling of contents and may introduce a sense of unfairness in the test taker. Choice items have gained popularity over the years in higher education. They can be developed relatively quickly and allow for the testing of a broad range of subjects in a short period of time. On the other hand, choice items have been criticized for being less flexible, mostly testing knowledge (memory) or knowledge application, which are the lowest levels of cognitive functions. Most important, scoring choice items is straightforward, unbiased, and rapid even when done manually. This provides a rich source of reliable information. The psychometric proprieties of choice items are important indicators of the reliability of the measurement and the discriminating power of the tool. With the advancement of computer technology, this statistical analysis has evolved from simple arithmetic as found in classical test theory (CTT) to sophisticated mathematics as found in item response theory (IRT) [30]. Although CTT is a deterministic model that provides measurements of the test performance as a whole and of the difficulty and discrimination power of individual items, it depends on the cohort of test takers and is based on the premise that items' characteristics are similar across the spectrum of performance, which is not true. IRT is a probability model that was developed to correct this by developing metrics that are independent of the population taking the test. It provides information that is intrinsic to the item ability as well as providing information about sources of error outside the domain of knowledge such as guessing. IRT allows for the development of adaptive test modalities such as computerized adaptive testing, which uses population independent statistics to provide a test form that is tailored to the test taker to maximize measurement precision [30].

Scoring test items is a critical step in the assessment process and is potentially a source of error. Traditional items have a relatively straight-forward process that can be fully automated as in choice items or that need the intervention of a judge to determine the extent of correctness in choice items. The emergence of machine learning, however, has provided tools to bridge best-of-choice and open-answer items. VSAQs are a simplistic form of machine learning with a scoring system based on a list of potential correct answers that can be matched to the answer given by the test taker. Its main limitations are the number of words that can be accepted (usually fewer than five) and the need for human decision when the inserted answer does not match the incorrect or correct list of options. Recent developments have further expanded this potential by using fully automated marking of open-answer and small narrative items. Using dictionaries of words and natural language processing, these computer algorithms can mark small pieces of narrative text with better precision than a human judge [31].

Score Reporting and Feedback Provision

Using two case studies, we now address the utility of technology in developing score reporting and feedback see **Case 7-1** and **Case 7-2**.

▌ HOW TECHNOLOGY IS IMPACTING OPERATIONS

Testing Modality (Adaptive Testing Models)

In computer-adaptive tests (CATs), an algorithm tailors a unique examination for each candidate to maximize the precision of measurement at his or her specific ability level with the fewest number of items possible. It does so by using IRT as a core model [30]. In one CAT scenario, the probability of a correct response is computed for an initial item of average difficulty using an IRT model. The candidate's answer to this item determines whether an easier or more difficult question is subsequently administered—that is, the examination "adapts" to the candidate's ability until precision of measurement can no longer be improved. Complementary to the gains in measurement precision, CAT needs a shorter period of assessment and a smaller number of items to estimate the candidate's ability. This represents an obvious gain in time but also reduces the number of exposed items because only a small fraction of candidates sees the same item, and each candidate has a specific set of items to which he or she is exposed. In addition, CAT has been shown to improve learning and may be a future form of adaptative assessment

---

Case 7-1: Reports as Student Feedback and Remediation Guides

Problem:

The director of a course on clinical skills wishes to provide feedback to students on an Objective Structured Clinical Examination (OSCE) test regarding three dimensions: clinical interview, physical examination, and planning. These placements vary in duration, and the moment within the course. How might the director provide meaningful and accurate feedback to students?

Solution:

The clinical skills course assesses learners through a series of 6 OSCE stations in three moments during the course. The assessment blueprint needs to be carefully designed so that each of the three dimensions is adequately sampled in each placement. The format of the OSCE stations should be homogenous to avoid presentation bias. Each station checklist must include items that are related to all dimensions in the blueprint but are specific to station content. For example, if the assessment outcome is the assessment of family history in one station the item would be "The student identifies mother had cancer?" while another station might be "The student identifies the father has diabetes?". This way the reporting of the general performance on family history taking can be reported without disclosing the checklist. This feedback can be used by students to improve specific dimensions in their clinical skills from one assessment moment to another.

Take Home message:

Careful planning of a blueprint and characterization of metadata is essential to ensure adequate sampling and data driven reporting to students. These reports are essential to allow students to reflect on specific aspects of their performance and search for remediation strategies.

---

and learning method [32]. Although CATs are attractive because they can yield precise measurements of abilities with shorter test lengths, especially large item banks are necessary to sustain such programs using sophisticated software packages [30].

Test Security

Test security is critical to ensure that the assessment process is fair and valid [33]. This is particularly important in high-stakes settings such as licensing

Case 7-2: Digital Score Reporting

Problem:

The head of assessment at a medical school wishes to report on scores of the progress test taken by students of all 6 years of a medical course. These happen every quarter within the course. How might learners be reassured that their scores are equivalent to the same standard and achieve the same learning outcomes?

Solution:

The progress test assesses all areas of the medical course through a combination of four blueprint dimensions: discipline (e.g., anatomy, cardiology, etc.), organic system (e.g., pulmonary, urinary, etc.), physician task (e.g., diagnosis, treatment), and cognitive task (e.g., memory, decision, etc.). Because students at different levels of development have different performances, raw scores would not be comparable among groups. To overcome this difficulty, scores should be reported based on reference to a norm. Adequate reporting should include information regarding each learner's position in the cohort performance curve with a visual depiction of the group's performance. Central and dispersion measures should be reported to each dimension of the blueprint. This way students understand their relative performance toward their own cohort and understand the relative difficulty of each area within the blueprint without disclosing any items.

Take Home Message:

Informative score reporting is critical for learners to understand their areas of strengths and areas to improve. Visual representation of the student's position in the cohort's performance makes it more tangible and relevant.

examinations and testing for competitive processes such as career choice. Although this has been a core issue in the assessment field, it remains secretive; many institutions withhold information on security breaches. So, it is unclear to which extent test security is a small or big concern.

CBT has improved testing security by reducing the number of intermediaries involved in the preparation and administration of tests. Establishing a direct link between servers in the licensing bodies and the test taker's computer enables higher protection. In addition, the use of security facilities with a controlled environment greatly reduces the chances of collusion and person-in-the-middle type of inter-ference. In addition, electronic assessment provides additional sources of information such as keystroke, mouse tracking, response times, and other parameters that relate to the test taker's behavior during the exam that can be used to analyze suspected security breaches in the postadministration period [34].

Item Review Processes

Item review is an essential step to ensure that test items have high qual-ity and provide accurate and reliable measurements of performance [35]. The establishment of item review committees has long been advocated. Licensing bodies such as certification boards and professional item devel-opers have dedicated teams to this task that thoroughly review items before administration. However, many small and middle-sized institutions struggle to implement them. This is partly because of the amount of time and resources that are needed to implement such procedures. Many soft-ware packages that are specialized in the assessment process now provide the possibility to develop item banks in a collaborative and hierarchical manner, thus providing an easier and less expensive way to implement item review committees. Moreover, the possibility to interact in a virtual nonsynchronous environment provides a chance for people from different geographical regions and time zones to collaborate in international proj-ects, something that would demand significant amounts of money and resources when done on-site. These online solutions typically provide a digital fingerprint to the entire development cycle of an item that can be used in auditing processes.

TECHNOLOGY IN ASSESSMENT—PROGNOSTICATIONS AND CONFABULATIONS

Assessment has advanced greatly in the last few decades. Computational capacity that was once reserved for big technological companies can now be achieved with a personal computer. In addition, open-source code and a growing number of data scientists have taken the ultimate step by democratizing computer programs that provide the tools for advanced assessment techniques. Artificial intelligence (AI) tools will become pro-viders of old and novel formats of assessment in a near future. Conversely, as we grow comfortable with the use of natural language processing and other forms of machine learning, we will be able to delegate traditionally human-dependent tasks such as scoring essays by computer. Eventually, this will free our time to gain efficiency—for example, by developing better

AIG models and developing novel forms of assessment such as a virtual patient encounter with real-life dialogues or computer-generated imagery for virtual patients. As data and knowledge grow, we will be able to produce better statistics and make better and faster decisions. It is likely that in a not-so-distant future, computers will be able to combine the automation of item generation and the application of adaptative processes on the fly. The exclusion of the human factor in the scoring could represent the fairest way to assess one's performance. This would represent the ultimate personalized, precise, and fairest assessment tool.

▌CONCLUSION

Human knowledge grows exponentially each year and will be accelerating with the dominance of AI. In the presence of *big data*, decision-making has become incredibly complex. It is impossible for professionals to cognitively contend with this complexity. The same holds true with assessment and measurement models. Current psychometric models do well with the kind of data we collect using traditional tools, but they do poorly with sparse and unstructured data. AI tools will potentially uncover data structures that humans simply cannot identify, which leads to new ways and systems for creating more authentic and complex learning and testing scenarios. Computer technology is not the problem. It is the solution.

The use of diagnostic, management, data mining, and summarization algorithms is already drastically altering education and assessment. The professional's role will be even more critical in regard to the introduction, evaluation, and best use of these technologies in their role as "advisor and knowledge navigator." AI and assessment will be a "team sport" predicated on a set of new competencies (statistics, computer sciences, etc.)

▌REFERENCES

1. Gier MJ, Lai H. Using automated processes to generate test items and their associated solutions and rationales to support formative feedback. *Interaction Design and Architecture(S)*. 2015;25(1):9–20.

2. Gierl MJ, Haladyna TM. Automatic item generation: An introduction. In: Gierl MJ, Haladyna, eds. *Automatic Item Generation: Theory and Practice*. Routledge; 2012. doi:10.4324/9780203803912.

3. Gierl M, Lai H, Hogan J, Matovinovic D. A Method for Generating Educational Test Items That Are Aligned to the Common Core State Standards. *Journal of Applied Testing Technology*. 2015;16(1):1–18.

4. Gierl MJ, Lai H. A Process for Reviewing and Evaluating Generated Test Items. *Educational Measurement: Issues and Practice*. 2016;35(4):6–20. Retrieved from https://doi.org/10.1111/emip.12129.

5. Gierl MJ, Lai H, Pugh D, et al. Evaluating the Psychometric Characteristics of Generated Multiple-Choice Test Items. *Applied Measurement in Education*. 2016;29(3):196–210. Retrieved from https://doi.org/10.1080/08957347.2016.1171 768.

6. Medrano LA, Liporace MF, Pérez E. Computerized assessment system for academic satisfaction (ASAS) for first-year university student. *Electronic Journal of Research in Educational Psychology*. 2014;12(2):541–562.

7. Gierl MJ, Lai H. The Role of Item Models in Automatic Item Generation. *International Journal of Testing*. 2012;12(3):273–298. Retrieved from https://doi.org/10.1080/15305058.2011.635830.

8. Kosh AE, Simpson MA, Bickel L, Kellogg M, Sanford-Moore E. A Cost–Benefit Analysis of Automatic Item Generation. *Educational Measurement: Issues and Practice*. 2019;38(1):48–53. Retrieved from https://doi.org/10.1111/emip.12237.

9. David MFB, Davis MH, Harden RM, et al. AMEE Medical Education Guide No. 24: Portfolios as a Method of Student Assessment. *Medical Teacher*. 2001;23(6):535–551. Retrieved from https://doi.org/10.1080/01421590120090952.

10. Gierl MJ, Lai H. Evaluating the Quality of Medical Multiple-Choice Items Created with Automated Processes. *Medical Education*. 2013;47(7):726–733. Retrieved from https://doi.org/10.1111/medu.12202.

11. Batalden P, Leach D, Swing S, Dreyfus H, Dreyfus S. General Competencies and Accreditation in Graduate Medical Education. *Health Affairs*. 2002;21(5):103–111. Retrieved from https://doi.org/10.1377/hlthaff.21.5.103.

12. Holmboe ES, Ward DS, Reznick RK, et al. Faculty Development in Assessment: The Missing Link in Competency-Based Medical Education. *Academic Medicine*. 2011;86(4):460–467. Retrieved from https://doi.org/10.1097/ACM.0b013e31820cb2a7.

13. Gierl MJ, Lai H, Turner SR. Using Automatic Item Generation to Create Multiple-Choice Test Items. *Medical Education*. 2012;46(8):757–765. Retrieved from https://doi.org/10.1111/j.1365-2923.2012.04289.x.

14. Royal KD, Hedgpeth M-W, Jeon T, Colford CM. Automated Item Generation: The Future of Medical Education Assessment? *EMJ Innov*. 2018;2(1):88–93.

15. McCoubrie P. Improving the Fairness of Multiple-Choice Questions: A Literature Review. *Medical Teacher*. 2004;26(8):709–712. Retrieved from https://doi.org/10.1080/01421590400013495.

16. Sinharay S, Johnson MS, Williamson DM. Calibrating Item Families and Summarizing the Results Using Family Expected Response Functions. *Journal of Educational and Behavioral Statistics*. 2003;28(4):295–313. Retrieved from https://doi.org/10.3102/10769986028004295.

17. Arendasy ME, Sommer M. Using Automatic Item Generation to Meet the Increasing Item Demands of High-Stakes Educational and Occupational Assessment. *Learning and Individual Differences*. 2012;22(1):112–117. Retrieved from https://doi.org/10.1016/j.lindif.2011.11.005.

18. Choi J, Kim H, Pak S. Evaluation of Automatic Item Generation Utilities in Formative Assessment Application for Korean High School Students. *Journal of Educational Issues*. 2018;4(1):68. Retrieved from https://doi.org/10.5296/jei.v4i1.12630.

19. Arendasy M, Sommer M. Using Psychometric Technology in Educational Assessment: The Case of a Schema-Based Isomorphic Approach to the Automatic Generation of Quantitative Reasoning Items. *Learning and Individual Differences*. 2007;17(4):366–383. Retrieved from https://doi.org/10.1016/j.lindif.2007.03.005.+

20. Gierl MJ, Lai H. Instructional Topics in Educational Measurement (ITEMS) Module: Using Automated Processes to Generate Test Items. *Educational Measurement: Issues and Practice*. 2013b;32(3):36–50. Retrieved from https://doi.org/10.1111/emip.12018.

21. Jozefowicz RF, Koeppen BM, Case S, et al. The Quality of In-House Medical School Examinations. *Academic Medicine*. 2002;77(2):156–161. Retrieved from https://doi.org/10.1097/00001888-200202000-00016.

22. Pugh D, De Champlain A, Gierl M, Lai H, Touchie C. Using Cognitive Models to Develop Quality Multiple-Choice Questions. *Medical Teacher*. 2016;38(8):838–843. Retrieved from https://doi.org/10.3109/0142159X.2016.1150989.

23. Blum D, Holling H. Automatic Generation of Figural Analogies with the IMak Package. *Frontiers in Psychology*. 2018;9:1–13. Retrieved from https://doi.org/10.3389/fpsyg.2018.01286.

24. Gunabushanam G, Taylor CR, Mathur M, Bokhari J, Scoutt LM. Automated Test-Item Generation System for Retrieval Practice in Radiology Education. *Academic Radiology*. 2019;26(6):851–859. Retrieved from https://doi.org/10.1016/j.acra.2018.09.017.

25. Lai H, Gierl MJ, Touchie C, et al. Using Automatic Item Generation to Improve the Quality of MCQ Distractors. *Teaching and Learning in Medicine*. 2016;28(2):166–173. Retrieved from https://doi.org/10.1080/10401334.2016.1146608.

26. von Davier M. Automated Item Generation with Recurrent Neural Networks. *Psychometrika*. 2018;83(4):847–857. doi:10.1007/s11336-018-9608-y

27. Cole BS, Lima-Walton E, Brunnert K, Vesey WB, Raha K. Taming the Firehose: Unsupervised Machine Learning for Syntactic Partitioning of Large Volumes of Automatically Generated Items to Assist Automated Test Assembly. *J Appl Test Technol*. 2020;21(1):1–11.

28. Sam AH, Field SM, Collares CF, et al. Very-Short-Answer Questions: Reliability, Discrimination and Acceptability. *Medical Education*. 2018;52(4):447–455. Retrieved from https://doi.org/10.1111/medu.13504.

29. Sam AH, Peleva E, Fung CY, et al. Very Short Answer Questions: A Novel Approach to Summative Assessments in Pathology. *Advances in Medical Education and Practice*. 2019;10:943–948. Retrieved from https://doi.org/10.2147/amep.s197977.

30. De Champlain AF. A Primer on Classical Test Theory and Item Response Theory for Assessments in Medical Education. *Medical Education*. 2010;44(1):109–117. Retrieved from https://doi.org/10.1111/j.1365-2923.2009.03425.x.

31. Latifi S, Gierl MJ, Boulais AP, De Champlain AF. Using Automated Scoring to Evaluate Written Responses in English and French on a High-Stakes Clinical Competency Examination. *Eval Health Prof*. 2016 Mar;39(1):100–113.

32. Martin AJ, Lazendic G. Computer-Adaptive Testing: Implications for Students' Achievement, Motivation, Engagement, and Subjective Test Experience. *Journal of Educational Psychology*. 2018;110(1):27–45.

33. American Psychological Association, American Educational Research Association, & National Council on Measurement in Education. *Standards for Educational and Psychological Testing*. Washington, DC: American Psychological Association; 2014. ISBN-10: 0935302352, ISBN-13: 978-0935302-35-6. Retrieved from https://www.aera.net/Publications/Books/Standards-for-Educational-Psychological-Testing-2014-Edition.

34. McManus IC, Lissauer T, Williams SE. Detecting Cheating in Written Medical Examinations by Statistical Analysis of Similarity of Answers: Pilot Study. *BMJ*. 2005;330(7499):1064–1066. doi:10.1136/bmj.330.7499.1064.

35. Wallach PM, Crespo LM, Holtzman KZ, Galbraith RM, Swanson DB. Use of a Committee Review Process to Improve the Quality of Course Examinations. *Advances in Health Sciences Education*. 2006;11:61–68.

8 Assuring Equivalence of Assessments across Settings

Tim J. Wilkinson and Vishna Devi Nadarajah

CHAPTER HIGHLIGHTS

- Equivalence of assessments is needed where assessments occur in different places or at different times.
- The focus should be on achieving equivalence of decisions rather than equivalence of assessment episodes.
- Standardizing assessments may or may not lead to equivalence. Moreover, it is only one way to ensure equivalence.
- Assessment organizers should devise ways to look for sources of bias that may undermine robust decisions. Differences between groups, however, do not always indicate presence of bias.

Scenario

A medical education program has learners studying the same program in many different locations. All have just completed a series of assessments that will determine eligibility to progress to the next year of the program. The learners in one center seem to have performed less well than the learners in the other centers, and they claim that the assessments therefore were unfair.

If you were the academic lead or coordinator for assessments, what would you do?

▌ ORIENTATION TO THE CHAPTER

Ensuring equivalence of assessments is a requirement of any system in which assessments occur in different places or at different times and where those assessments are used to inform high-stakes decisions. Examples include medical school assessments across different clinical sites, medical school assessments occurring at different times, postgraduate assessments across different clinical sites, selection assessments occurring in several countries, learners wishing to transfer between programs who have undertaken all previous assessments in a different program, and national licensing assessments. When differences are found, learners may take the view that the assessments were unfair, but there are many other possible explanations as to why the learners may not have done so well. This chapter aims to help a reader understand some of these issues and to look at quality measures that could be put in place to try to avoid, or at least explain, any perceived problems with unfairness.

INTRODUCTION—WHY MIGHT WE WANT EQUIVALENCE?

Assessments are often used to inform whether someone has learned enough; this could be to decide whether the person gains a qualification, is permitted to proceed into a job, or is ready to proceed to the next stage of training. In these circumstances, it is implicit that such judgments are being made against a standard. Alternatively, assessments can be used to rank learners; this applies particularly in situations where there are limited opportunities to proceed to the next stage such as competitive entry situations where there are more applicants than positions. In both circumstances (assessment against a standard or assessment for limited opportunities) assessment is of the individual's learning. Here learners would wish to be reassured that such judgments are robust and independent of when, where, or how the assessment took place.

However, we also know that assessment drives learning and can be used to inform where learners might next best place their efforts. In these circumstances, where we are using assessment primarily to be *for* learning rather than *of* learning, achieving equivalence is often not needed. This chapter focuses on situations in which assessment is used to inform high-stakes decisions and aimed primarily around assessment of learning.

UNDERSTANDING EQUIVALENCE

We begin by asking what do we mean by ensuring equivalence of assessment across settings? *Equivalence*, *fairness*, *validity*, and *lack of bias* are inter-related terms. In all cases, the goal is for an assessment to reflect what a learner has learned. Ideally, learners who have achieved the intended learning outcomes to similar levels should achieve at the same levels on assessments. This refers to validity—the extent to which the assessments assess what is intended to be assessed. Anything contributing to the result that is unrelated to learner achievement—such as where, when, or how the assessments occurred—also contributes to a lack of equivalence. Furthermore, anything that threatens the ability to achieve such equivalence undermines the validity of both the assessment process and decisions arising from that process. Likewise, if there are learners who truly differ in capabilities but seem to achieve similar assessment scores, this also undermines the validity of the assessment process. Assessment decisions should assess the true learning of the learners, regardless of where or when the assessments took place. Assessments that are not valid are unfair.

At this point, it is important to explain what is meant by learners who truly differ in a meaningful way. A common pitfall is to look at assessment results and feel reassured if we see a broad range of scores. Some examiners feel similarly falsely reassured if the scores they give show a good spread across test takers. This is simplistic because even random sampling will produce a range of scores. In contrast, an assessment designed to look at mastery of an area should not necessarily produce a range of scores; there should only be results that separate those who have mastered the area from those who have not. So our question should always be, do our results differentiate between the learners who have achieved the intended outcomes from those who have not? In the case of selection for limited places (for example, entry to medical school or job applications), the question should be, do our results differentiate between those who are best suited to be admitted compared with those who are not?

In broad terms, differences in assessment results could arise from true differences between learners, differing perceptions of the expected standards by examiners, some problems with administration of the assessments, or differences in curriculum delivery in a particular setting. If the assessments occur across national or cultural boundaries, then any differences in performance between learners might also be explained by differences in regulatory requirements or differences in sociocultural understandings of what is expected. See **Cases 8-1** and **8-2**.

Why are these issues important? Clearly, the learners worry about them as they become concerned that their true performance is not reflected in the assessment decisions. Our stakeholders also worry about this because they wish to be reassured that the standards we set for our learners are maintained equitably across all settings. For example, if the learners from one setting are less able compared to those from another but this is not reflected in their assessment outcomes, then a stakeholder might question the robustness of the process. Historically, many have felt reassured that if the reliability of the assessment is of sufficient standard, then such concerns regarding equivalence or unfairness are unfounded. It's not that simple, and this chapter aims to outline some of the issues that should be considered.

Case 8-1: Assessments across Different Clinical Sites

Problem:

The first 3 years of a medical course occur for all learners in one city, but the later years of the course place learners in several different cities. These placements vary in nature, duration, and the year within the course. How might the public be reassured that the learners all graduate to the same standard and achieve the same learning outcomes?

Solution:

The medical course assesses learners through a combination of in-course Work Based Assessments (WBAs) and end-of-year examinations. These examinations are identical for all learners, regardless of the city in which they are placed. The assessment blueprint, however, shows that not all learning outcomes can be assessed through these examinations, so equivalence in the in-course assessments also needs to be shown. Any learner who performs below an expected standard on the in-course assessments is discussed by a competence committee, one for each city. These committees also bring the details of learners for whom they have remaining concerns to a joint meeting where they are discussed by representatives from all cities. In this way, problem sharing and the more important discussion about these learners contribute to shared understanding of the expected standards while also ensuring that all learners who pass have met the same common standard.

Take Home Message:

Learning opportunities can vary according to where learners are placed. Quality assurance of how the learning outcomes have been achieved can be attained though clear blueprinting of the suite of assessment tools. Conversations among faculty members can be an effective mechanism for shared understanding of the expected standards. The goal should be competence or fitness to practice regardless of setting while making best use of local experiences, opportunities, and constraints.

Case 8-2: Learners Transferring between Medical Programs

Problem:

International medical programs have been designed to meet the needs of stakeholders in a global setting [1]. The model for international medical programs sometimes requires students to have learning experiences and assessment decisions in one country and then transfer to other countries to complete their medical degrees. The stakeholders for these types of programs would, for example, include international and home students, institutions receiving the students or transferring the students out, and clients and patients in both countries. How would institutions as stakeholders ensure acceptance and equivalence in the assessment outcomes despite variations in the assessment settings?

Solution:

The solution to this case study is similar to that for **Case 8-1**. For example, there needs to be a general agreement of the expected learning and assessment outcomes before the students transfer to the receiving international partner institution. Assessment best practices such as blueprinting, vetting, standard setting, and assessor training should also be made transparent across institutions to ensure that good practice is implemented and evaluated from time to time. At the International Medical University (IMU) in Malaysia, which has a medical program that partners with more than 20 medical schools abroad, additional measures such as faculty training with partner schools' assessment experts and inviting external examiners from partner schools on a rotating cycle for progression point assessments to help ensure the stakeholders of practices that will enhance equivalence. At IMU, there are yearly meetings with representatives from all the partner schools called the Academic Council in which all matters related to quality assurance, including assessments measures, for transfers are jointly discussed. These yearly joint discussions are opportunities to continuously enhance the partnership and ensure acceptance

Take Home Message:

Institutions as stakeholders in international partnerships need to continuously work toward a shared understanding of standards and governance procedures. Regular structured, open, and transparent communications on issues such as assessments are opportunities to continually enhance the partnership and ensure acceptance to the broader stakeholders such as students, regulators, and patients.

Equivalence Versus Standardization

A simplistic way of thinking we might have achieved equivalence is to look at the reliability of our assessments. If the reliability is above a predefined standard, then we might regard the assessment as being of sufficient quality. This is a simplistic approach and does not recognize many of the other factors that could affect how learners might perform on an assessment other than those related to their true ability. Another simplistic way of reassuring ourselves regarding equivalence of assessment is to make sure that all the assessments are completely standardized. Standardization means that the assessments are identical, often simultaneous, and administered in an equal way across all settings. The problem with standardization or overemphasis on reliability is that they often threaten authenticity [2]. The types of assessments that can be administered in a standardized or highly reliable way tend to be quite limited; as a consequence, they tend to be unable to assess all the attributes we regard as important. National examinations are an example of this. Such examinations tend to be restricted in format often because of logistic limitations. For example, a national examination commonly uses the Multiple Choice Question (MCQ) format. Although there are many important attributes that can validly be assessed using MCQs, many attributes are less able to be assessed in this way. Examples include collaboration with others, communication skills, and performance under pressure. Ironically, it is these same attributes that are less able to be assessed in this way that are often more highly valued by our stakeholders: Not everything that counts can be counted [3].

To some readers, it may seem counterintuitive that not all assessments need to be reliable. Increasingly, concepts of reliability extend beyond individual assessment events or individual examinations. Instead, the aggregation of several pieces of unreliable information, if synthesized and interpreted in an appropriate way, can lead to highly reliable decisions [4,5]. To use a clinical analogy, if we were to assess whether a person might be in heart failure, we could just rely on the height of the jugular venous pressure. However, we know that the inter-rater reliability of such measurements is not high. Likewise, the presence or absence of a third heart sound can be helpful but also has low inter-rater agreement. Should we therefore disregard such assessments? If we assimilate and synthesize all of these pieces of information, including other assessments such as symptoms and changes in body weight and then pull these pieces of information together, we can often arrive at a reliable decision. Unreliable assessments should not be disregarded, but neither should high-stakes decisions be made on them alone. Instead, deferring a decision until there is sufficient information can make best use of all available data while maintaining reliability and validity. This is the philosophical underpinning of programmatic assessment [6].

Taking this approach can free us from the concerns of *unstandardized* assessment tools (such as those that require use of real patients) or even *unstandardized* assessors. Provided the results from enough assessment episodes and enough examiners are synthesized, then reliable decisions can be reached—often with greater validity [4].

When the Objective Structured Clinical Examination (OSCE) was first established, it was thought that its reliability came from the standardization of the tasks and from the use of standardized checklists (see **Case 8-3**). As already indicated in **Chapter 4**, we now understand that the reliability of an OSCE comes not from the overspecification of the task but from the aggregation of the information from all stations. Each station on its own is often

---

Case 8-3: Inter-rater Agreement on Checklist versus Global Scores

Problem:

In a high-stakes OSCE, two examiners are assigned to assess each test taker on each station. Although the OSCE's overall internal consistency was good (around 0.8), the inter-rater agreement between pairs of examiners varied. The organizers of the OSCE concluded this was the result of insufficient details in each station about what should be assessed.

Solution:

The organizers tried to remedy this by making the checklist items in the marking schedule more specific. This also resulted in an increased number of checklist items. What the organizers found in doing this was no benefit on inter-rater agreement [7,9]. Instead, the examiners found the marking tasks more challenging because they had to spend more time looking at the checklists than taking a broad view of how each test taker was performing. The change annoyed the examiners and provided no additional benefit on *objectivity*.

Take Home Message:

Agreement on global scores is often as good or even better than agreement on checklists—provided the examiners have a shared understanding of what is valued. Too many checklists risk trivializing the task [2]. Differences between examiners are less critical than ensuring each test taker is seen by enough examiners—that way, the aggregate view of all examiners provides a good picture of each test taker.

unreliable, but the aggregation of many such stations leads to a reliable decision. Likewise, we have come to realize that reliability can be just as high, if not higher, from global ratings by examiners than from overspecified checklists [7] (see **Case 8-3**). Reliability comes not purely from objectivity but from multiple collective views, the so-called subjective collective [8].

In other words, reliability not only comes from standardization but also is often better achieved when there is adequate sampling, robust synthesis of information, and rigorous interpretation. The reliability of the decision becomes more important than the reliability of each individual source of data.

However, even here there can be threats to the reliability of such decisions. If the individual assessments have not been conducted appropriately or if the understanding of the agreed standard differs according to the decision-makers, then less fair decisions can arise.

CONTRIBUTORS TO LEARNER ASSESSMENT RESULTS

Table 8-1 shows examples of contributors to a learner assessment result. Each will be discussed in the following sections.

Learner Factors

Learners' Actual Learning

What the learner has actually learned is the factor that we most want to represent in any assessment result. In other words, the test results should be higher for those learners who truly have learned than for those who have not. Alternatively, we do not always want a grade or numerical score, in which case the goal here is that the learners who pass the assessment should be those who are suitable to progress to the next stage of training and the learners who fail are not yet ready to proceed.

Sometimes we want our assessment results to reflect learner ability or future potential—that is, more able learners scoring higher than less able learners. Here it is important to distinguish between a learner's inherent ability and what they have learned. In general terms, our education programs are designed to help learning, so assessments during or after such programs aim to determine what has been learned. However, some assessments are undertaken in order to select those who are most suitable for a training program, in which case the assessments here are designed more to assess a person's potential rather than what they have learned to date. In either case, determining what a learner has learned or what his or

Table 8-1   EXAMPLES OF CONTRIBUTORS TO A LEARNER ASSESSMENT RESULT

Learner Factors
- Learner's actual learning
- Background factors that might lead to bias (e.g., gender, language, ethnicity, country of origin)
- Impairment—permanent or temporary
- Performance anxiety
- Test "wiseness"

Administrative and Technological Issues
- Assigning learners to assessment groups or times of the day on the basis of identification number or in or alphabetical order
- Type of device
- Data capacity and bandwidth

Teaching and Learning Factors
- Differences in curriculum learning opportunities
- Availability of examination preparation material

Policy Factors
- Adherence to agreed processes

Assessment Factors
- Assessment tool authenticity
- Construct validity and sampling
- Item construction, particularly any bias introduced by language or cultural differences
- Reliability
- Differences in administration
- Security
- Standard setting

Examiner Factors
- Degree of shared understanding of assessment purpose
- Degree of shared understanding of expected standards of performance
- Similarities or differences between the examiner and the learner
- Inattention
- Prior knowledge of other aspects of a learner's performance

Decision-Making Factors
- Degree of shared understanding of assessment purpose
- Degree of shared understanding of expected standards of performance
- Bias from synthesizing multiple pieces of information
- Bias from group decision-making

her potential might be becomes the aspect of assessment that we wish to maximize and other sources of variation in scores should be minimized.

Learner Background

Learners' assessment results might be affected by their backgrounds—for example, gender, first language, ethnicity, or country of origin. In general, such differences raise the possibility of unwanted bias. However, interpretation of such differences needs to consider the purpose of the test because any observed differences might not always be the result of bias. For example, consider a test designed to determine a learner's ability to communicate. Test takers whose first language is different from the test language may perform less well on the test. Where language proficiency is a prerequisite for good communication, such a result might be a desired outcome of the test rather than showing bias against test takers who have a different first language. Likewise, a test might be designed to determine if test takers are able to understand the cultural norms of the people with whom they will interact. In this case, if test takers from a different culture perform less well on the test, this may not always indicate bias but might indicate a lack of learning of test takers from a particular background. In any case, any differences on assessment scores that seem to relate to a test taker's background need to be considered and explained, considering the purpose of the assessment, rather than automatically being dismissed as bias or true differences.

Impairment

Test taker impairment is often a cause for people to do less well on tests. Here again, interpretation of any variation from the expected result needs to consider the purpose of the assessment under question. For a test taker with a temporary impairment (e.g., a broken arm), the challenge becomes determining how that test taker might have performed had that impairment not been present. One way to do this would be to ask the test taker to defer sitting the assessment until the impairment is no longer present. Often this is not feasible for practical reasons, so judgments need to be made. Sometimes extra assistance to overcome their impairment may be needed while at other times an adjustment in the score might need to be considered. All these decisions require careful consideration, judgment, and justification, but the goal is to determine how that test taker might have performed had the impairment not been present (see **Case 8-4**).

The situation of a permanent impairment (e.g., dyslexia) raises extra issues to be considered. The key question here becomes what is the likely impact of that permanent impairment on the future performance of the

Case 8-4: Driving a Car Versus Becoming a Histopathologist

Problem:

A person requires spectacles to correct his or her vision and wishes to drive a car. In taking the driving test, the use of special assistance (spectacles) would be appropriately permitted during the assessment. This is because it could be reasonably expected that the same assistance would be available when undertaking the task authentically. In fact, it might be a requirement that such assistance is used when the assessment was undertaken under those circumstances.

A person is color blind and wishes to become a histopathologist. In this job, visual interpretation of color stains in histological preparations is an essential component. During the assessment, no amount of extra assistance or adjustment of any assessment score is likely to validly represent that learner's ability to perform that job in the future [10].

Solution:

Providing extra assistance or adjustments needs to consider both the nature of the impairment and the nature of the tasks that passing the assessment would allow a person to undertake. Some assistance may undermine validity by concealing a person's true ability. Some assistance may enhance validity by allowing a person's true ability to be more apparent. In some cases, the provision of assistance may have implications for how or if a person is permitted to perform in a specific job.

There might be some permanent impairments that impact a person's ability to undertake the assessment but not his or her ability to undertake a job in an authentic situation. This might be where the assessment requires the test taker to undertake tasks that would not reasonably be expected in a workplace. A simple example could be typing skills versus handwriting. Consider a situation in which a test taker has an impairment that impacts handwriting but not typing. If the future job does not require handwriting skills, only typing skills, yet the assessment only permits handwritten answers, then assistance with handwriting to complete the assessments would be appropriate. Alternatively, arrangements could be made to allow the test taker to type answers to assessment questions.

Take Home Message:

The presence of an impairment does not automatically mean that extra time, special assistance, or adjustment of marks are needed. Instead any impact on the score from an impairment needs to be considered in relation to the purpose of the assessment and whether or not the impairment reduces the validity of any decision arising from that assessment. Measures to manage potential influences of impairment should be available and applied consistently at all sites where learning and assessment take place.

learner? For example, some permanent impairments will impact on the ability of a learner to perform the job that the education program is preparing them for. If, once in that job, no extra time, assistance, or compensation is available, then the assessments should also be undertaken without extra time, assistance, or compensation. In contrast, if it might reasonably be expected that help would be available for the person once in the job, then such help should be provided to undertake the assessments. Refer to **Case 8-4**.

Performance Anxiety

Any assessment is designed to make inferences about a learner's ability to perform in more authentic situations. If factors are present at the time of the assessment that would reasonably be expected to be absent in a more authentic situation, then these relate more to the assessment than to the attribute being assessed. As such, these are potential sources of bias or threats to validity. One example of this is performance anxiety under assessment circumstances. Such anxiety can sometimes be hard to interpret. For example, if a learner is expected to perform under pressure in an authentic situation and if the assessment reproduces that pressure, this is not necessarily a source of bias. However, if the source or the nature of the pressure in an assessment situation is sufficiently different from the nature of the pressure in a more valid situation, then this can be a source of bias. Furthermore, anxiety is not always the result of assessment alone. The learner who is worried about his or her ability can sometimes feel anxious, in which case the anxiety relates more to the lack of preparation and not necessarily to extraneous sources of bias. It goes without saying that unnecessary sources of pressure in an assessment situation should be eliminated, but any anxiety displayed by a test taker requires interpretation because it may or may not be contributing to the validity of the assessment outcome. As for the many examples given in this chapter, we need to ask whether the test conditions reflect or extrapolate to the job conditions?

Test Wiseness

As already discussed in **Chapter 3**, test wiseness can be an additional source of bias, this time to the advantage of some learners. This is where a learner's result on a test relates more to the test format than to what the test is designed to assess. For example, when the options on a multiple-choice test show some grammatical inconsistency, this can mean the correct answer is identified simply by a test taker's knowledge of grammar. If the test is designed to assess something else, then such grammatical flaws undermine the validity of that test item. They unfairly advantage test takers with attributes that were not designed to be part of the assessment process. To minimize bias from test wiseness, and as part of the quality assurance of assessments, item-writing training sessions, peer review, and standardization of assessment items or instructions across sites is necessary.

Administrative and Technological Issues

The actual implementation of assessments can vary in ways that may unexpectedly impact performance. An example is the order in which learners are assessed in an OSCE; examiner fatigue may impact test takers assessed later in the day, whereas question and station familiarization may affect how examiners mark learners earlier in the day. Often such effects are overstated, but being aware of these issues and looking for any source of bias related to test taker order or other administrative variations can be part of quality assurance processes.

Increasingly, many assessments rely on technology. Written tests can be conducted online in which test takers type their answers or provide answers to MCQs by computer. Likewise, and as learned during the COVID-19 pandemic, video-conference assessments are sometimes used to assess patient interactions or presentations skills. In many ways, these tests have similar authenticity to those taken without using technology. However, the addition of technology can add a risk if there are variations in data capacity or bandwidth or if test takers have inequitable access to appropriate devices [11]. For further details on the role of technology in assessment, please see **Chapters 7** and **10**.

Teaching and Learning

Test takers might perform better on an assessment simply because they received better teaching. This does not mean that the assessment is flawed. If the assessment accurately represents what learners have learned, then arguably the assessment is performing as expected. Learners might claim that the process is unfair, but in this case such unfairness is not the result of the assessments.

If there is inequitable availability of examination preparation material, then this can undermine the validity of the assessment because performance on the assessment might relate more to the availability of such material than to what the learner has learned. A common example of this is the "black market" of recalled test questions that some learners have access to and some others do not. Ideally, these learner-driven resources are available at all sites. Although this may be difficult for program leaders to control, this should be a topic that is discussed in regular learner–faculty meetings. Another example might be extra coaching that is only available for those learners who can afford it.

Policy Factors

We cannot expect all assessments to be standardized or to be identical, but we can expect that assessments might be undertaken under agreed situations and under agreed policies that govern assessment in all sites. Evidence that these policies are implemented is important for continuous quality improvement. When audits or learner appeals pick up missing documentary evidence of policy implementation, accreditation or non-compliance issues may follow. Learner appeals are most likely to be successful when such policies have not been followed or show inconsistencies between sites.

Assessment Factors

Determination of the equivalence of assessments should always be preceded by ensuring that the assessments themselves are of good quality. It is beyond the scope of this chapter to outline all the principles of good assessment, but in general anything that undermines the validity of an assessment will also undermine achievement of equivalence.

Good assessment always starts with ensuring validity. There should be content validity whereby the program of assessments reflects that which is expected to be learned; this is addressed through program-level blueprinting, which should be common across sites. *Construct validity* refers to the degree to which an assessment or assessments accurately measure what they are designed to measure. To do this, a clear description of the attributes being assessed should be given, and assessment events should aim to be samples of those attributes. It is rarely possible to assess all the attributes in depth. Instead, a judicious sample of such attributes should be undertaken. This often starts with blueprinting [12]. The next stage requires a choice of appropriate assessment tools, which ideally should be as authentic to the task as possible while balancing this with feasibility.

Care should be taken in item construction in order to avoid inadvertent bias. For example, if the people developing test items are not demographically or culturally representative of test takers, then bias can be introduced through cultural oversights that may disadvantage test takers who are not demographically similar to the item writers.

A reliable assessment does not guarantee equivalence, and assessments can also be reliable without being valid. Nevertheless, if a test is unreliable,

Case 8-5: Assessments from Home and Across Various Time Zones

Problem:

The issue of assessments across various time zones is not something new in medical education. Professional postgraduate assessments and selection examinations that cater to international test takers are often conducted across various time zones in different test centers across borders. The recent experiences with COVID-19 highlighted the need to conduct undergraduate assessments within a medical school both from home and in various time zones for cohorts with international students. How can medical schools adapt and administer the usual on-campus assessments to online home-based assessments in varying time zones in a fair manner?

Solution:

The shift to online assessments requires clear communications on the electronic devices, Internet capacity, and settings required for online assessments. A preassessment survey on the technological accessibility detailed in the communication will help administrators devise student support measures and guidelines for implementation. If there are instances in which students are unable to have stable Internet connection or a conducive home environment, arrangements can be made for students to have on-campus accessibility or use facilities in other partner institutions.

For students who are in time zones different from the main campus or central test administration sites, clear and early communications on the timings (campus time versus student local time) for assessment is needed. It is good administrative practice to request an acknowledgment of receipt on examination timings from these students. Having the assessments done concurrently across various time zones is preferred to avoid assessment security issues like cheating, which will affect the equivalence of assessments and should always be minimized.

Take Home Message:

The expected pass standard should be the same regardless of where a learner undertakes an assessment. Pass standards should normally be set so that they are applicable to all administrations of an assessment. If the purpose of an assessment is to determine competence, then standard setting should be criterion referenced. If the purpose of an assessment is to rank people, then norm referencing is often needed.

it becomes harder to ensure equivalence. As previously mentioned, reliability is not the function of a single test event but is often better achieved using multiple assessment events over time and making decisions on the synthesis of those results rather than on single assessment episodes.

Differences in administration of an assessment event can influence equivalence. For example, an examination might be identical in two places, but differing test-taking circumstances can affect the results. Simple examples include differences in the time given to take the test, the materials available to use, and extraneous factors such as noise or distractions. If the time of the test administration differs, then this can raise risks regarding examination security if it is possible for test takers who have just sat the test to communicate with test takers who are yet to sit it (see **Case 8-5**).

Examiner Factors

No matter how hard we try, differences between examiners in what they are looking for and how they mark a test taker will always exist. To some extent, this can be mitigated through examiner training and calibration, but a degree of subjectivity will always remain. Indeed, subjectivity is often what is asked for from examiners because they are asked to make judgments, and this can never be an automated or algorithm-driven process. The best way to improve the reliability of examiner judgments is to ensure that we do not rely on single judgments alone when making high-stakes decisions. Just as the reliability of a test is improved if we use multiple samples of a learner's ability, so too the reliability of examiners is improved if we ensure there are multiple examiners. This is often more fruitful than trying to focus too much on the performance of single examiners.

Nevertheless, some key factors can be ensured that will maximize the reliability and validity of examiner judgments. This starts with making sure all examiners understand the purpose of the assessment. For example, the purpose of some assessments might be to identify those learners who are yet to meet the minimum standard required to proceed to the next part of the course. For other assessments, it could be to discriminate among learners for ranking purposes. First, problems can arise if the examiner's view of the assessment purpose differs from the institution's view of the assessment purpose. Second, examiners need a shared understanding of the expected standard of performance. For example, examiners accustomed to assessing learners at a postgraduate level might apply unduly harsh judgments if they are assessing learners at an undergraduate level.

Examiners should be aware of conscious and unconscious sources of bias. A common source of bias arises from the degree of similarity between an examiner and a test taker. If the examiner and test taker share demographic similarities, then it becomes more likely that the examiner might favor that learner.

If an examiner is required to assess multiple learners at one time at one sitting, being tired or inattentive can introduce bias. Ensuring examiners have adequate breaks can mitigate this.

If an examiner has some prior knowledge of other aspects of a learner's performance, then this can introduce bias [13]. It is not always possible for test takers to be assessed by people they have never seen, but it is important for examiners to recognize that the judgment of a learner's performance at the time of an assessment could be influenced by what he or she knows about the test taker from other observations of his or her performance. Such variation could go either way—prior knowledge may influence an assessor to unduly pass or fail the test taker.

Although there is controversy over the effectiveness of examiner training [14,15], anyone's performance can improve after feedback. As such, providing feedback to examiners on their assessment ability can be a useful quality-improvement measure. However, simply comparing examiners by their mean scores or their spreads of scores can be misleading. Use of statistical techniques such as use of *item response theory* (IRT) models or generalizability studies [16–18] can separate out the contributions to a learner's score according to item quality and examiner factors. A focus on individual assessment items and individual examiners can sometimes be helpful, but it is also important to note that it is the quality of the overall assessment program rather than individual assessment items that is the most important. As previously outlined, the use of unreliable assessment items can still lead to reliable decisions provided enough items and enough examiners are used.

Decision-Making Factors

Once all the assessments have been undertaken and all information about a given learner is available, this information needs to be aggregated and synthesized to inform a robust decision. As for examiner decisions at the time of an assessment event, decision-making can also be prone to bias. More robust decisions are often made by a group of people rather than a single individual, but even group decisions can be subject to bias [19]. Examples include a dominant personality who overly influences the group and all members of a group thinking in the same way without the opportunity to challenge (*groupthink*). Decision-makers can also be unduly influenced if they personally witnessed one aspect of a learner's performance because this can have greater salience compared with all the other observations that the decision-maker did not witness. A personal anecdote can sometimes carry more weight than it should when compared with the aggregated information from all the other observations [20]. Making decisions on deidentified learners can often mitigate these risks.

As for examiner decisions, group decision-making also starts with making sure everyone understands the purpose of the assessment and having a shared understanding of the expected standard of performance. Quality is often enhanced if there is a designated person in the decision-making group who has the task of ensuring due processes are followed.

AVOIDING PITFALLS TO ACHIEVE EQUIVALENCE

Having looked at the various contributions to a lack of equivalence, we now turn to consider ways in which equivalence could be achieved. These are summarized in Table 8-2 and will be discussed.

Administer the Same Examination

A simple, and relatively common, way to achieve equivalence of assessments is to make them simultaneous and identical. All test takers sit the same examination at the same time. This achieves equivalence but provides a significant threat to examination authenticity and validity because not all attributes of importance can be assessed using such methods. For example, with regard to clinical exams, it may be difficult to ensure the similar case mix and complexities across the various settings.

Sometimes test takers could sit the same assessments but at different times. Unless there are mechanisms to prevent communication between test takers, this can cause problems related to examination security.

Use the Same Examiners

Having the same examiners mark all assessments can lead to better consistency. This is more feasible for written assessments. For practical or clinical assessments, this is sometimes achieved by using traveling examiners in which the same examiner assesses subsets of test takers from different sites. As previously mentioned, there can be variation in marks attributable to an examiner that can be difficult to differentiate from any variation in marks because of case difficulty or clinical scenario. This means that any similarities or differences found by a

Table 8-2 METHODS TO ACHIEVE EQUIVALENCE		
Method to Achieve Equivalence	**Advantage**	**Disadvantage**
Administer the same examination	Simple to achieve	Limits what can be assessed
Use the same examiners	Achieves consistency	Does not eliminate bias related to an examiner. Increased cost and time in travel to sites
Use the same questions or test items	Can be used to compare standards across test administrations	Risk of contamination from recalled or leaked questions that are reused (this can be mitigated if the item bank is large enough
Use equilibrated questions or test items	Can be used to compare standards across test administrations More efficient use of questions and test taker time. Lessens risk of leakage of questions for subsequent cohorts	Requires availability of statistical and technical assistance. Less applicable to nonwritten assessments
Attend to quality assurance of questions or test items	Can assist in identifying sources of bias and in identifying suitable marker questions	Requires access to psychometric expertise
Ensure the same high-stakes decisions would be taken when the assessment results are similar	High value for learners and stakeholders	Requires quality assurance processes to ensure consistency
Same processes for governance	Allows flexibility in timing and nature of assessment events	Requires documentation of and adherence to quality assurance processes

traveling examiner can be hard to interpret. Nevertheless, the face valid-ity of having a traveling examiner can be reassuring for learners and other stakeholders.

Rather than examining a subset of learners, another examiner could reassess a subset of question responses. This is sometimes called *moderation*, and it is often used for those questions or learners who are on the cusp of failing or passing. Having such questions remarked by an independent examiner can be one way of ensuring the robust-ness of such high-stakes decisions. Some institutions may video record a clinical encounter and view such recordings for moderation purposes.

The evidence for the effectiveness of examiner training is scant [14,15]. All examiners should have a shared understanding of the purpose of the assessment and of the expected standard, which training can address to some extent. In the case where an examiner is found to be consistently severe (a "hawk") or consistently lenient (a "dove"), it is less clear whether feedback from such performance alters subsequent behavior.

Use the Same Questions or Test Items

Rather than administering the same examination to all learners, it is sometimes more feasible to include a subset of questions to determine equivalence. Psychometric techniques and the availability of psychomet-ric expertise can be especially helpful here, although even simple statistical comparisons of item performance across sites can be useful. Such *marker questions* can be used between years to check if standard setting is being maintained or could be used between courses as a form of benchmark-ing [21]. One problem with reusing the same questions between the years is that questions can be remembered by test takers and communicated to subsequent cohorts. Such questions when reused this way might increasingly be answered correctly with repeated administrations, making the questions appear easier or the test takers appear more able over time.

Use Equilibrated Questions or Test Items

Under classical test theory, an item answered correctly by many test takers could reflect the item's lower level of difficulty or the test takers' higher levels of ability. Use of more sophisticated statistical analysis of ques-tions such as IRT models [18] can separate out difficulty from ability and thereby lead to better equilibration of questions.

One consequence of this is the opportunity to use computer-adaptive examinations where all questions have associated data on their perfor-mance metrics, particularly their difficulty. An estimate of a test taker's ability is obtained from the first set of questions answered, and those test takers with an estimated higher ability are given more difficult questions whereas those test takers with an estimated lower ability given easier questions until a stable measure of test taker ability is obtained. This means not all learners answer the same questions the same way. The length of the test can vary between test takers because those who have a stable measure of ability determined earlier can have a shorter test. The advantages of this approach are that it leads to more efficient use of questions, greater reliability using fewer items, and more efficient use of test taker time. All test takers do not answer the same questions or in the same order, so this reduces the leakage of questions for subsequent cohorts. Equivalence of standards across test takers and across years can be demonstrated more robustly.

Attend to Quality Assurance of Questions or Test Items

Questions answered incorrectly by most test takers could reflect test takers' low ability, the difficulty of the question, or an item-writing flaw. Quality assurance of questions can help, particularly use of IRT.

Some questions may not perform as expected and might contain inadvertent bias whereby some cultural, linguistic, and socioeconomic subgroups might be unfairly advantaged or disadvantaged. Ways to avoid this are to have questions reviewed by experts trained in identifying cultural bias or by representatives of culturally and linguistically diverse subgroups or to include more *performance-based* test formats to limit the role that language and word choice plays in test performance. Vetting of exam questions prior to exams can also be useful, particularly if examiners from various sites are involved. Quality assurance processes also extend to post hoc item analysis, which provides transparency for any moderation actions that might be needed.

Ensure the Same High-Stakes Decisions Would Be Taken When the Assessment Results Are Similar

We already know that there is considerable variation in assessment performance related to the item or to the examiner. For assessments that include patients or performance in the workplace there is a variation inherent in case specificity whereby performance is related to the nature of the patient's problem rather than just test taker ability. For WBAs contextual factors can also be considerably variable. It is neither possible nor desirable to standardize for all these factors. We also know that more reliable and robust decisions arise from the synthesis of multiple pieces of information on multiple occasions from multiple examiners. For the learner and for our stakeholders it is the decision that needs to be robust more than all the assessment items that lead to that decision. Scrutiny of decisions therefore is more likely to be fruitful in ensuring equivalence than too much scrutiny on individual assessment items. This means that some measure of the reproducibility of decisions is likely to be both robust and reassuring in ensuring equivalence of standards. For example, would a different set of decision-makers come to the same decision given the same set of assessment results for each learner? Alternatively, for those learners who have yet to reach the required standard to progress, or for those learners who have only just reached the required standard to progress, would a different set of decision-makers come to the same decision? While these are questions that assessment organizers should consider, the ways in which they could be answered may vary according to the context.

In this way the focus becomes on the system of assessment rather than the individual assessment items [22].

Same Processes for Governance

Documentation of and adherence to assessment processes can aid equivalence. Having visiting examiners oversee assessment processes is likely to be useful. Such visiting personnel could sit in at the time that an assessment is blueprinted, be part of any standard-setting process, or sit in when pass–fail decisions are being made. Input into these aspects can be one way of providing reassurance that processes are being adhered to and followed, with some benchmarking to practices in other institutions.

❚ WAYS TO MEASURE OR EVALUATE EQUIVALENCE

When looking at assessment results, the primary question we must answer is, are the results as we might expect? We then should look at different cohorts of learners and decide if the similarities or differences between cohorts are as we might expect.

Learners can be divided into groups in many different ways. We could divide them according to the site of administration of the assessments or according to their backgrounds. Likewise, the assessment results can be subdivided in many different ways. We could look at the results according to the mode of assessment such as the type of tool used (e.g., MCQ versus OSCE). We could also look at the assessment results according to the type of the attribute being assessed. All these comparisons have the potential to find differences, many of which can be informative. However, there is also a real risk of a type 1 error whereby significant differences are found purely by chance. When this occurs, there is also a risk of overinterpretation and undue anxiety.

In contrast, there is a risk of underinterpretation of results if a cursory look shows no apparent differences between cohorts. This is because

> ## Case 8-6: Cohort Performance Trends over Time
>
> ### Problem:
>
> In 2010 and 2011, a series of earthquakes in Christchurch, New Zealand, disrupted medical learners' education, disrupted health services, and closed the main medical school building for 2 years. However, the medical course was still delivered, largely as planned. The question was asked whether this had an impact on learner performance and whether this differed from the cohort of learners in two other cities who were less impacted by the earthquakes and sat the same examinations.
>
> ### Solution:
>
> It was possible to use learner results from earlier in the course to see how well they predicted results later in the course. It was then possible to use this model to determine if there was any differential effect on the learners in Christchurch. In fact, a large earthquake that was close to the time of the end-of-year examinations did have a measurable effect, but a more devastating earthquake some months before the end-of-year examinations did not. [23]
>
> ### Take Home Message:
>
> It is possible to look at a cohort's prior performance to determine if apparent differences between cohorts could be explained by factors other than the assessment itself.

actual differences between cohorts have been concealed through insufficient analysis. This might create undue complacency.

As a result, it is better to look at trends over time and repeated differences between groups rather than to place too much concern over apparent one-off differences (see **Case 8-6**).

Interpreting assessment results is most easily done if there are some other measures of learner learning other than the assessment results themselves. This way, these other measures can be compared with assessment results to see if they show associations that might be expected. One simple example of this is to compare learners' current assessment results with their results from previous assessments. In general, one might expect learners who have performed well on assessments in an earlier year to perform well on assessments in subsequent years, assuming that the assessment tools are designed to assess similar attributes. Likewise, if the assessments have been specifically designed to look at different attributes from previously, then one might expect to find lesser association.

There is not always a clear relationship between the attribute being assessed and the format of the assessment. For example, MCQs do not just test knowledge and OSCEs do not just assess skills. Instead there might be components within each format or modality of assessment that might be expected to correlate. For example, a test taker's knowledge of pediatrics might correlate with their clinical skills in pediatrics. One way therefore of exploring the validity of a suite of assessments is to see whether the correlation between attributes is higher than between modalities of assessment. Even here, however, interpretation can be difficult.

Exploring any differences according to the examiner can be more problematic unless each learner has been examined by more than one examiner at the same time. In such cases, one can look at simple inter-rater correlations. However, one needs to be aware that two examiners can have a high inter-rater correlation yet still not mark equivalently. For example, if examiner A consistently marks 5% higher than examiner B, then the inter-rater correlation will be high but their inter-rater agreement will be low. Some comparison of means or measures of absolute agreement may also therefore be necessary. There are inter-rater agreement indices that take these absolute differences also into account. For clinical assessments, interpretation of examiner results can be more problematic because it is not uncommon for an examiner to examine only a subset of all learners; when a patient is part of the assessment, the learner result may depend as much on the patient as on the examiner. Provided the learner result is taken by aggregating all examiners and all patients, this usually does not cause any systematic bias or lack of equivalence. There are statistical techniques— for example, generalizability theory—that can determine how much of score variance might come from the learner, the patient, or the scenario being examined, or from the examiner [24]. Determining whether any variance results from examiners might be attributable to a single person can be more difficult unless trends over multiple occasions can be explored.

Interpretation of any assessment differences according to learner attribute requires considerable interpretation. For example, finding a difference in learner performance according to ethnicity does not automatically mean that bias is present without considering other confounding variables. Nevertheless, if one assessment shows a difference but all other assessments show no difference according to ethnicity that cannot otherwise be explained, then there should be scrutiny into that assessment to look for any sources of systematic bias.

Table 8-3 outlines some suggested quality measures that could be used to determine the standardization or equivalence of assessments.

Table 8-3   EXAMPLES OF QUALITY MEASURES THAT COULD ENSURE STANDARDIZATION OR EQUIVALENCE OF ASSESSMENTS

Assessment Purpose
- The purpose of the program of assessment is stated
- The purpose of each assessment event is stated
- The purpose is the same across test administrations

Learning Outcomes
- The learning outcomes that could be assessed are known to the learners
- There is a process to ensure sufficient sampling of a learner's performance from those learning outcomes at the program level
- There is a process to ensure sufficient sampling of a learner's performance from those learning outcomes at the assessment event level.
- The mechanism to decide sampling (blueprinting) is the same across assessment event administrations
- The mechanism to decide sampling (blueprinting) is the same across the various assessment sites

Standard Setting
- There is a process for ensuring standards are understood by examiners and that this is the same across assessment event administrations and sites
- There is a process for ensuring the pass standard is set for any assessment event
- Pass standards are the same across test administrations and, where appropriate, over time.

Decision-Making
- The processes for decision making are documented
- High-stakes decisions are reliable by ensuring they are informed by sufficient samples of a learner's performance and by a sufficient number of different examiners
- Decisions are made on de-identified learners
- Decisions are made by a group

Bias
There are processes to identify or minimize sources of bias in
- test or assessment event format
- item construction
- test or assessment event construction
- examiner scoring,
- decision making
- administration site

Test or Assessment Event Evaluation
- There is periodic evaluation of assessment item performance according to learner subgroups
- There is periodic evaluation of test/assessment event performance according to learner subgroups
- There is periodic comparison of results from assessments to determine if assessments that are designed to assess the same attributes are correlated better than assessments that are designed to assess different attributes

▌CONCLUSION

The first step toward determining whether there is equivalence of assessments is to recognize that there is the potential for factors other than a learner's true ability to affect how they perform on an assessment. The second step is to systematically look for evidence of any such lack of equivalence and take measures to avoid it. Having learners sit the same assessments at the same time can create equivalence, but this also threatens the quality of the program of assessment. Instead, the focus should be on ensuring that learners are assessed using multiple formats, over multiple occasions, with a range of examiners ensuring sampling from a well-constructed blueprint against the desired learning outcomes. Equivalence of decisions is more important than equivalence or standardization of assessment episodes. Evaluation of a program of assessment should explore evidence for any systematic bias and ensure that well-documented policies are followed.

▌REFERENCES

1. Brouwer E, Driessen E, Mamat NH, et al. Educating Universal Professionals or Global Physicians? A Multi-Centre Study of International Medical Programmes Design. *Medical Teacher*. 2020;42(2):221–227.
2. van der Vleuten CPM, Norman GR, De Graaff E. Pitfalls in the Pursuit of Objectivity: Issues of Reliability. *Medical Education*. 1991;25(2):110–118.
3. Wilkinson TJ. Pass/Fail Grading: Not Everything That Counts Can Be Counted. *Medical Education*. 2011;45:860–862.
4. Schuwirth LWT, van der Vleuten CPM. Programmatic Assessment and Kane's Validity Perspective. *Medical Education*. 2012;46(1):38–48.
5. Wilkinson TJ, Campbell PJ, Judd SJ. Reliability of the Long Case. *Medical Education*. 2008;42(9):887–893.
6. Schuwirth LWT, Van der Vleuten CPM. Programmatic Assessment: From Assessment of Learning to Assessment for Learning. *Medical Teacher*. 2011; 33(6):478–485.
7. Wilkinson TJ, Frampton CM, Thompson-Fawcett MW, Egan AG. Objectivity in Objective Structured Clinical Examinations: Checklists Are No Substitute for Examiner Commitment. *Academic Medicine*. 2003;78(2):219–223.
8. Hodges B. Assessment in the Post-Psychometric Era: Learning to Love the Subjective and Collective. *Medical Teacher*. 2013;35(7):564–568.
9. Wilkinson TJ. How Not to Put the O into an OSCE. *Perspectives on Medical Education*. 2018;7:28-29.
10. Spalding JAB, Cole BL, Mir FA. Advice for Medical Students and Practitioners with Colour Vision Deficiency: A Website Resource. *Clinical and Experimental Optometry*. 2010;93(1):39–41.
11. Er HM, Nadarajah VD, Wong PS, Mitra NK, Ibrahim Z. Practical Considerations for Online Open Book Examinations in Remote Settings. *MedEdPublish*. 2020; 9(1):153.

12. Er HM, Nadarajah VD, Chen YS, et al. Twelve Tips for Institutional Approach to Outcome-Based Education in Health Professions Programmes. *Medical Teacher*. 2019:1–6.

13. Stroud L, Herold J, Tomlinson G, Cavalcanti R. Who You Know or What You Know? Effect of Examiner Familiarity with Residents on OSCE Scores. *Academic Medicine: Journal of the Association of American Medical Colleges*. 2011;86:S8–S11.

14. Fryer G, McPherson HC, O'Keefe P. The Effect of Training on the Inter-Examiner and Intra-Examiner Reliability of the Seated Flexion Test and Assessment of Pelvic Anatomical Landmarks with Palpation. *International Journal of Osteopathic Medicine*. 2005;8(4):131–138.

15. Newble DI, Hoare J, Sheldrake PF. The Selection and Training of Examiners for Clinical Examinations. *Med Educ*. 1980;14(5):345–349.

16. McManus IC, Thompson M, Mollon J. Assessment of Examiner Leniency and Stringency ('Hawk-Dove Effect') in the MRCP(UK) Clinical Examination (PACES) Using Multi-Facet Rasch Modelling. *BMC Medical Education*. 2006;6:42.

17. Bloch R, Norman G. Generalizability Theory for the Perplexed: A Practical Introduction and Guide—AMEE Guide No. 68. *Medical Teacher*. 2012;34(11):960–992.

18. De Champlain AF. A Primer on Classical Test Theory and Item Response Theory for Assessments in Medical Education. *Medical Education*. 2009;44(1):109-117.

19. Hauer KE, Cate OT, Boscardin CK, et al. Ensuring Resident Competence: A Narrative Review of the Literature on Group Decision Making to Inform the Work of Clinical Competency Committees. *Journal of Graduate Medical Education*. 2016;8(2):156–164.

20. Tweed MJ, Thompson-Fawcett M, Wilkinson TJ. Decision-Making Bias in Assessment: The Effect of Aggregating Objective Information and Anecdote. *Medical Teacher*. 2013;35(10):832–837.

21. Wilkinson TJ, Hudson JN, McColl GJ, et al. Medical School Benchmarking—From Tools to Programmes. *Medical Teacher*. 2015;37(2):146–152.

22. Norcini J, Anderson MB, Bollela V, et al. 2018 Consensus Framework for Good Assessment. *Medical Teacher*. 2018;40(11):1102–1109.

23. Wilkinson TJ, Ali AN, Bell CJ, Carter FA, Frampton CM, McKenzie JM. The Impact of Learning Environment Disruption on Medical Student Performance. *Medical Education*. 2013;47(2):210–213.

24. Crossley J, Davies H, Humphris G, Jolly B. Generalisability: A Key to Unlock Professional Assessment. *Medical Education*. 2002;36(10):972–978.

Quality Assurance of an Assessment Program 9

Lonneke L.H. Schellekens, Bert Slof, and Harold G.J. Bok

CHAPTER HIGHLIGHTS

- Practical design guidelines for ensuring a program's assessment
- Case study quality assurance; blueprint assessment policy plan
- Case study quality assurance; tool visualizing and monitoring assessment quality
- Theoretical perspectives on developing quality-assured assessment programs

ORIENTATION TO THE CHAPTER

This chapter starts with an introduction of procedures and methods for ensuring the quality of an assessment program in practice. Two case studies will be presented to enhance understanding of how these procedures and methods can be applied to educational practice. Because different quality perspectives on assessment programs exist, insight will be provided into the continuum of theoretical perspectives of program's assessment quality by offering some rules of thumb (i.e., quality indicators) and associated quality assurance procedures. The chapter will end with concluding remarks and present do's and don'ts to avoid common pitfalls.

INTRODUCTION

Educational programs in many fields are often aimed at selecting or qualifying learners for future educational programs and jobs [1–3], so it is important to know whether learners have actually sufficiently mastered the required knowledge, skills, and attitudes. To establish this, programs should at least assess whether their learners have met required proficiency levels in a summative manner (e.g., pass–fail decision). How programs organize this (e.g., viewpoint, choices, and operationalization) is often explicated in their assessment programs [4,5]. We regard an assessment program as a mix of various assessment methods that are deliberately composed and appropriate for the aims, content, and structure of the curriculum [6,7].

Having a sound assessment program is vital for a wide range of stakeholders. It could enhance the transparency of the assessment (e.g., goal, type, number, pass score) for its learners. In addition, it could support teachers, program directors, and examination boards in discussing and aligning the (course-specific) assessments. Furthermore, it might provide employees an indication of what they can expect from the program's alumni. Although this sounds promising, the presumed beneficial effects for educational and workplace-related practices strongly depend on the quality of the assessment program. More specifically, the stakeholders need to gain insight into what the underlying quality indicators and procedures are and how these procedures are properly utilized.

▌ASSESSMENT PROGRAM'S QUALITY IN PRACTICE

Quality and Quality Assurance of an Assessment Program

Quality assurance of an assessment program addresses the question of how the quality of a program is guaranteed [8]. To guarantee the quality of an assessment program, in practice three interrelated aspects of quality are often distinguished [9–11]:

1. a focus on quality as input, associated with how the program is designed;
2. a focus on quality as output, associated with insight into and examination of clearly defined and structured learning outcomes, and the extent to which set goals are achieved;
3. a focus on quality as a process, associated with procedures that monitor, manage, and evaluate the desired effect of plans and actions for improvements consequent to assessment.

The three aspects can function as guidelines to assure assessment quality at the program level.

Quality as Input: Design of an Assessment Program

The assessment program is part of the overall learning process [6]. To highlight the functionality of assessment for student learning, it is important that the assessment process is carefully designed [12]. The design of the assessment program should be properly aligned with the program's educational philosophy. A well-functioning assessment program that supports learning and ensures high quality decisions [6,13,14] includes:

- alignment of assessment, learning activities, and learning outcomes within and throughout the program;
- content that covers and contributes cumulatively to the educational outcomes;
- both formative and summative assessments as appropriate to its purposes;
- effective and efficient use of resources; and
- transparent and acceptable procedures and results that address the multiple needs of the educational stakeholders and future employees.

The starting point of the design of an assessment program is to determine the purpose of the program. An often-used criterion that reflects a program's quality in this stage is "fitness for purpose" [12], which refers to "the extent to which a program of assessment fulfils its purpose or its function" (p. 2), indicating that assessment activities should be designed congruent with the rationale that is reflected in the purpose. Subsequently, the purpose determines how the guidelines to design an assessment program are considered. These guidelines are formulated with regard to the core activities of the program and the way these can be optimized; how the organizational learning is captured and how the program of assessment can be improved; and how evidence can be provided that the purpose of the program is achieved [12].

Quality as Output: Learning Outcomes

Learning outcomes describe the final qualifications of a study program and refer to specific levels of knowledge, skills, or ability for a given profession. At the individual student level, learning outcomes are used to express what learners are expected to achieve and how they are expected to demonstrate that achievement [15]. At the program level, outcomes are more broadly defined as development or growth, representing what the educational program aims to teach its students and what the labor market can expect from its alumni [16]. Assessing and demonstrating the achievement of these outcomes is important for connecting higher education with the larger society. By demonstrating how the learning outcomes are achieved, insight is given in the alignment of teaching with the learning outcomes, which ensures the validity of the degree awarded to the student [16]. Evaluation of the structure of learning outcomes and how they are assessed throughout the program is also important to foster dialogue, review, and justification within the program [16,17].

Learning outcomes can be informed or directed by career requirements, and professional or accreditation standards. Although individual programs determine their own version of general educational outcomes, there are some (inter)national models that can provide guidance. For example, medical curricula tend to identify competency domains or roles as areas specific for the profession in which students need to develop their performance in meeting societal needs—for example, the CanMEDS framework [18]. In the Netherlands, the VetPro competency framework consists of 16 competencies organized around seven domains, which a graduate veterinary specialist should be able to fulfil [19]. The initial rationale for these frameworks was to provide (inter)national recognition for academic degrees. However, by providing broad descriptors of learning outcomes, these frameworks also provide potential reference points for external quality assurance practices [20].

At the moment, indicators of student learning outcomes as part of the quality assurance process framework have become prominent in many countries, including the United States, Australia, New Zealand, the United Kingdom and South Africa [11]. Quality assurance denotes the practices whereby learning outcomes, i.e., the level of academic achievement attained by higher education graduates, are maintained and improved [20]. To evaluate learning outcomes at the program level, institutions must collect evidence about student skills, competences, and abilities to prove that the program-level outcomes or goals are achieved. Evidence may embrace the results of both quantitative and qualitative data [11]. As the contexts of higher education and the practices of implementing learning outcomes differ a lot, no one single method for the implementation and evaluation of achieved learning outcomes exists [16]. However, when the quality of an assessment program is not reviewed at the program level, the use of learning outcomes is not easily monitored.

Quality as Process: Internal and External Procedures

A quality assurance system may utilize measures of academic quality by means of internal and external assurance procedures. "Internal quality assurance" refers to those policies and practices whereby educational institutions themselves monitor and improve the quality of their education provision [20]. Internal quality assurance comprises for example monitoring and analyzing student assessment scores and evaluations, and self-evaluation procedures [10,21]. In addition, to ensure that courses are effective in the longer term, graduates' experiences and employers' perceptions are needed for the improvement of programs [17]. Self-evaluative procedures can be a good preparation for accreditation and are seen as an effective approach to both ensure external quality assurance and increase internal quality [8]. Moreover, self-evaluation not only results in concrete points for improvement, but is also good to raise awareness among the educational stakeholders [22].

An example of an effective self-evaluation procedure was recently developed by Sluijsmans and colleagues [8]. Their method—"the assessment assessed"—motivates programs in taking more responsibility and autonomy in processes that assure educational quality. The method distinguishes five phases in the development of assessment quality that indicate how assessment stakeholders are oriented within the assessment process. Program directors and teachers are asked to self-assess the current and desired position, for example with regard to an assessment task or -program. These insights can help to formulate improvement actions that are necessary to achieve the desired position. The following developmental stages were distinguished. Stakeholders can be oriented on:

1. separate ad hoc activities which are carried out by individual stakeholders in the study program;
2. the process in which relevant stakeholders in the study program carry out assessment activities based on a short-term policy;
3. the system by which all relevant stakeholders in the study program are oriented toward a medium-term policy and activities are interrelated and integrated into ongoing processes in practice;
4. a chain in which all relevant stakeholders in the study program pursue a medium-term policy together; oriented with chain partners, assessment activities are interrelated and integrated in ongoing processes in practice and the chain;
5. a society in which all relevant stakeholders in the study program pursue a long-term policy; together with oriented chain partners and society, assessment activities are interrelated and integrated in current processes in practice and the chain and society.

Another example of a self-evaluation procedure on program level is developed by Baartman and colleagues [21,23,24]. They proposed a framework of 12 quality criteria based on psychometric and edumetric criteria that can be used formatively to evaluate the quality of competence-assessment programs.

"External quality assurance procedures" refers to external policies and practices that assure the quality of an institution or study program [20].

External quality assurance is often provided by an external auditing committee—for example, in an accreditation of a program for authorization or certification. In an accreditation process, criteria and standards are formulated as a benchmark against which the program will be assessed [10]. External assurance can also be provided by giving information to external stakeholders—for example, to inform student choice by means of outcome measures such as graduate placement and salaries [20,25]. These latter indicators of quality increasingly have been published by government and academic institutions to better inform student choice because education has become more competitive nationally and internationally [20]. An important debate, therefore, in quality assurance is whether the purpose of external evaluations is aimed at accountability or improvement [9]. The European University Association [9] argues that the introduction of internal quality procedures can serve as a balance to the requirements of external accountability. Nevertheless, in Europe, quality assurance has tended to focus on measurement and standards. For example, the alignment of standards with goals of summative assessment, rather than on aspects of assessment that improve student learning [26].

Reflection on Quality Assurance in Practice

To guarantee the quality of an assessment program, the focus should always be at all three aspects—input, output, and procedures—because these refer to a continuous and iterative process of monitoring, analysis, and action [10]. The various assessment stakeholders—students, teachers, and future employees—should be involved and be part of quality assurance procedures to review and renew the curriculum. This requires a coherent quality management system that facilitates dialogues between the stakeholders and that provide insight into the curriculum and its quality [6]. The overall aim is to establish a quality culture that encompasses the whole institution in a consistent manner, reflected by educational enhancement that is based on the experiences, expertise, and values of the institute [9].

In the next sections, two case studies (**Case 9-1** and **9-2**) are presented that show how the guidelines are implemented in practice. The first case study describes an example of quality assurance by implementation of an assessment policy plan. By applying high-quality standards (i.e., psychometric and edumetric criteria) and related procedures in the policy plan, the risk of making incorrect decisions (e.g., false positive or false negative) can be minimized [5,27]. This gives internal stakeholders (e.g., students, teachers, and examination boards) the confidence that the assessments are carried out in a responsible manner; consequently, a signature can be placed under the diplomas with confidence. It also provides external stakeholders (e.g., labor market, accreditation organizations) insight into why the program meets national or international standards. The second case study refers to a tool that is developed to visualize and monitor assessment quality at both the course and program levels. By giving insight into assessment quality, the tool aims to support continuous improvement by enabling dialogues between assessment stakeholders and by facilitating an effective the plan, do, check, act (PDCA) cycle [8,28].

CASE 9-1: ASSURANCE BY ASSESSMENT POLICY PLAN

Program Description and Identified Problem

The Faculty of Social & Behavioural Sciences at Utrecht University in the Netherlands focuses on the disciplines of interdisciplinary social sciences, cultural anthropology, educational sciences, pedagogy, psychology, and sociology. The faculty offers bachelor's, master's, and PhD programs and has around 850 employees and more than 5,600 students. The directors of the bachelor's and one-year master's programs of the Faculty of Social & Behavioural Sciences have written their assessment policy plans since 2014. These policy plans are annually commented on, rewritten, and discussed with the faculty's examination board. Furthermore, the policy plans are used to inform accreditation commissions about the program's assessment policy (quality indicators, procedures, assurance).

Although valuable, in recent years most policy plans turned into documents consisting of 60 or more pages (e.g., describing each course in detail), which jeopardizes its usability (e.g., lacking an overview at the program level and constructive discussions). Two main reasons for this were (1) a lack of clarity about what had and had not been described within each section and (2) the (experienced) perception that the plans should be written for accountability purposes only. This is unfortunate because, on the one hand, the policy plans are an important benchmark for accreditation commissions and examination boards. On the other hand, they could also provide valuable input for constructive discussions about assessment quality both within (e.g., teaching staff, examination board) and between (e.g., program directors, vice deans) educational programs. With the aim of improving the usability of the assessment policy plans, the faculty's examination board developed a new template for the program directors. By doing so, the experienced "bulkiness" and lack of clarity associated with the previous policy plans can hopefully be reduced and the plans become a more integral part of the educational programs.

Reasons for Change

Providing good-quality education is of paramount importance to all educational programs and society. Each program should, therefore, strive to offer a program in which students work in an active, differentiated, and challenging manner on achieving the (personalized) training objectives. To realize this, the three pillars of constructive alignment [13] are utilized in an integrated manner:

1. Learning outcomes—What does the program aim to teach its students?
2. Content and structure of the program—How will the program teach its students, and so on?
3. Assessment—How does the program assess whether its students achieve the educational objectives?

In the policy plan, the psychometric and edumetric quality assurance demands were therefore addressed in an integrated manner using the interpretative argument approach ([29,30], see also "Continuum of Theoretical Perspectives on Assessment Program's Quality." This means that the (1) learning outcomes (section 1), (2) educational program (section 2), and (3) assessment policy (section 3) are drawn up in an integrated manner. Furthermore, the procedures for monitoring the quality requirements at the course, program and faculty level should be described (section 4). Noteworthy to mention here is that the policy plan consists of a fixed format with predefined texts that have been tailored (i.e., checking if the predefined description fits or should be adjusted) to the program's specifications.

Designed Assessment Program

Learning Outcomes

Defining and substantiating the learning outcomes is the starting point for the assessment policy plan. The learning outcomes define how broadly or specifically the program intends to profile itself and how this relates to the (inter)national standards and labor market (see Table 9-1). In Europe, the Bologna Process resulted in a common framework for higher education wherein five main learning outcomes of all degrees are described, the so-called Dublin Descriptors [11]. Therefore, in Dutch higher education, the profiling is usually based on the European standards (i.e., Dublin Descriptors) as well as the domain-specific frame of reference that outlines the field of study in relation to the labor market.

Program directors are requested to briefly (in a maximum of a single page) substantiate their choice for the selected learning outcomes.

Table 9-1	OVERVIEW OF LEARNING OUTCOMES IN RELATION TO THE DUBLIN DESCRIPTORS (DD)	
Dublin Descriptors*	**Label**	**Learning Outcomes**
DD1 Knowledge	DD1_1	
	DD1_2	
	...	...
DD2 Application and insight	DD2_1	
	...	...
DD3: Judgment	DD3_1	
DD4 Communication	DD4_1	
DD5 Learning Skills	DD5_1	
	...	...

*DD1: Knowledge; DD2 = application and insight; DD3 = judgment; DD4 = communication; DD5 = learning skills

By doing so, they provide various stakeholders (e.g., students, teachers, examination board) insight into the extent to which the learning outcomes align with:

- the domain-specific frame of reference (external factors),
- what the program believes can be expected from their alumni (internal factors), and
- the Dublin Descriptors and whether they can be obtained within the available number of credit points.

Educational Program

The learning outcomes are the starting point for shaping the educational program—namely, providing the subject matter in a logically structured manner. The development of learning tracks is a means for providing insight into and justifying the content and structure of the program [31,32]. A learning track is often defined as a specific focus area (i.e., combination of courses) for which the outcomes, subject matter, and didactics have to be related in an orderly (e.g., structure in complexity) and responsible manner. It is important that the choice for the learning tracks and their interplay are described in a transparent manner. By doing so, the program can ensure that the students are able to obtain the learning outcomes.

Designed Educational Program

Program directors are requested to provide a brief overview (maximum of two pages) of the selected learning tracks (see Table 9-2) and provide in each track a brief description of associated courses, learning outcomes and mastery levels, and subject matter.

Substantiation of the Educational Program

Program directors are requested to briefly (maximum of one page) substantiate their choice for the interplay between the selected learning tracks. By doing so, they provide various stakeholders (e.g., students, teachers, examination board) insight into the extent to which the learning tracks:

- can be distinguished from another in terms of the subject matter taught,
- are built up (within and between) in a coherent manner (i.e., subject matter, outcomes, mastery level), and
- enable students to obtain all of the program's learning outcomes.

Assessment Policy

With the learning outcomes and the educational program as a starting point, the subsequent assessment policy will be drawn up [22]. The assessment policy should describe a well-balanced mix of the (1) assessment methods (including weighting and content coverage), (2) assessment moments (planning, re-sit opportunity), (3) consequences (formative

Table 9-2	OVERVIEW OF LEARNING TRACKS AND COVERAGE OF LEARNING OUTCOMES					
Learning Outcomes						
DD 1	DD 2	DD 3	DD 4	DD 5	Courses	Learning Track*
					1 …	A
					2 …	
					3 …	
					…	
					…	…

*Learning track A

and summative), and (4) granularity (ratio group and individual assessment).

Design Assessment Policy

Program directors are requested to provide a brief overview of assessment policy (see Table 9-3) by describing per learning track, the:

- type of assessment instrument(s) and their granularity (individual or groupwise) that are administered, and
- the instruments that will be administered to assess intended learning outcomes.

Substantiation of the Assessment Policy

Program directors are requested to briefly (maximum of one page) substantiate their choice for the assessment policy. By doing so, they provide various stakeholders (e.g., students, teachers, examination board) insight into the extent to which the:

- learning outcomes are assessed in a summative as well as a formative manner,
- instruments are suited for assessing the learning goals (including mastery level),
- assessments are administered in a reliable manner,

Table 9-3 OVERVIEW OF ASSESSMENT POLICY							
Assessment		**Learning Track**[**]	**Learning Outcomes**				
Instrument	**Granularity**[*]		**DD_1**[***]	**DD_2**	**DD_3**	**DD_4**	**DD_5**
Exam		A					
Paper							
Thesis							
Practicum							
Presentation							
...							
...		..					

[*]Ratio (%) per assessment instrument, indicating whether it is administered individually or groupwise.
[**]Learning track A
[***]Dublin Descriptor 1

- scoring criteria and grading procedures are transparent for all involved stakeholders, and
- the weighing and granularity of the instruments are appropriate for assessing whether each individual student obtained the program's learning outcomes.

Quality Assurance Procedures

An important goal of the assessment policy plan is that the examination board can confidently sign the degrees. To this end, the board member must trust the procedures that are utilized to ensure that the learning outcomes are taught and assessed properly. In addition to utilizing the constructive alignment principle, this requires continuous monitoring and, if required, the refinement of the psychometric and edumetric quality demands. The quality assurance procedures are utilized according to the PDCA cycle [8,28] and involve an interplay between three different levels.

At the *course level* the coordinators utilize several procedures to ensure high assessment quality. For the psychometric quality demands, an assessment plan (i.e., substantiated overview of the course learning outcomes and associated assessments) and an assessment matrix (i.e., substantiated overview of a specific assessment's items and associated mastery levels) are drawn up. For the edumetric quality demands, the course coordinators utilize several procedures aimed at increasing the transparency of the assessment to all involved stakeholders. For example, students have the opportunity to practice (e.g., mock exam, concept paper, thesis) so that they can receive feedback on their performance before it is assessed summatively.

At the *program level*, the director is the linking pin between the different courses as well as the program's assessment policy and the faculty's and university's assessment policy. The director is responsible for the assessment policy plan and its implantation into the different courses. Usually this is done by having regular and constructive discussions with the responsible course coordinators. The policy plan also serves as input for discussing the quality assurance procedures at the faculty level (e.g., annual interviews, quality assurance interviews). Course and curriculum evaluations are administered, and the findings are used as input for refining the course and the assessment policy plan. Furthermore, the director makes inquiries about training needs.

At the *faculty level*, various activities are carried out to ensure the assessment quality—that is, policy documents (e.g., education and examination regulations) are drawn up and provide directions for the assessment at the program and, consequently, the course level. The faculty's examination board is an active and independent committee that moni-tors the utilization of the quality assurance procedures and intervenes (e.g., constructive feedback, mandatory adjustments) when required at all levels. The board reports annually to the faculty management. If neces-sary, the responsible vice dean can use this information during the annual quality assurance meetings with the program directors. In these meetings, several aspects of the assessment quality are discussed, namely (1) coher-ence, structure, and diversity of the assessment; (2) alignment of learning outcomes and assessment; and (3) quality assurance procedures utilized at the program and course levels.

Outcomes and Lessons Learned

By implementing a faculty-wide program assessment policy, a general framework including associated guidelines for all stakeholders is pro-vided. This should support stakeholders at different organizational levels (i.e., dean, program director, exam committee teachers, students) in the development and implementation of an educational program in which the program learning outcomes and structure as well as the assessment are properly aligned. Note that programs should also have some degrees of freedom in determining how they want to align things. Based on the sug-gested rules of thumb, educational programs can tailor the framework to their own characteristics and discuss their choices with other stakeholders such as the faculty's exam committee.

CASE 9-2: ASSURANCE BY USING AN TOOL: E-QUALITY

Program Description and Identified Problem

Educational programs often encounter difficulties in enhancing an assess-ment culture and ensuring assessment quality. For many programs it is challenging to facilitate an effective PDCA cycle because information about the quality of the entire assessment process, both on a course and curricu-lum level, tends to be scattered around a large group of stakeholders. In response, the application E-quality was developed at Utrecht University in the Netherlands. It offers educational programs the opportunity to sus-tainably enhance and ensure the quality of their assessment program. It provides a gateway to document and visualize all activities performed in relation to assessment quality on a course and curriculum level. By creat-ing a dashboard accessible for all relevant stakeholders (e.g., teachers, edu-cational management, and examination board), the application provides a transparent overview of current assessment quality and supports continuous improvement. It aims to foster a productive dialogue between all stakeholders to discuss a school's current assessment quality and formulate objectives for improvement. In addition, the application facilitates the collection of assessment information over multiple years, demonstrating structural quality improvement for accountability issues.

Currently, E-quality is being tested in a pilot experiment at three different educational programs at Utrecht University. For the development of this pilot version of the application, different stakeholders were involved. Among others, teachers, educational directors, and examination board members with a background in a variety of curricula and different assessment strategies (e.g., traditional summative approaches, programmatic approaches) provided input in the development of the final version to be piloted. The results of this pilot will be used to improve the usability and efficiency of the application. To learn about what does and does not work in practice, scientific research is conducted to evaluate its impact on the assessment quality and assessment culture. In an iterative process of design, implementation, evaluation, and redesign, the application is continuously improved to best accomplish its goals in sustainably improving the quality of assessments.

Reasons for Change

What do we understand by improving the assessment quality? And what is a better assessment culture? Many educational programs formulated in their strategic plans the ambition to establish a culture that is focused on improvement. Just like learners, all stakeholders involved in the educational journey require feedback on their performance to promote self-directed learning. With respect to assessment, this "feedback" relates to the different aspects involved in sustainably enhancing and monitoring the assessment quality. To sustainably improve the assessment quality, E-quality adopted a programmatic approach toward assessment. Please see **Chapter 6** for details on programmatic assessment. High-quality assessment (from students to management) is characterized by having an assessment culture focused on learning. Therefore, at a course level, the application provides opportunities for assessors to reflect on current assessment practices and formulate new goals to improve performance. At the same time, the increased insight in assessment quality fosters continuous dialogue between different stakeholders about the organization's assessment ambitions, the current state of assessment quality, and realistic short- and long-term measures to improve assessment quality. In creating a clear and compact overview of all relevant assessment information, the application provides evidence for accountability issues—that is, program accreditation. Through the adoption of this approach, improving quality will become an integral part of daily educational practice and help programs sustainably create a culture that is intrinsically focused on improvement.

As a foundation for E-quality, the quality criteria of an assessment program described by Baartman [23] combined with the work done by Sluijsmans and colleagues [8] were used to develop a beta version. Based on a first pilot study with teachers, educational directors, and examination board members, further adjustments and refinements were made to optimize the formulation and relevance of the quality criteria. The following criteria to ensure assessment quality are included in the application at course and program levels: learning impact, reliability, validity, and transparency (see Box 9-1 for a description).

Designed Assessment Program

To sustainably improve assessment quality, the application aims to effectively visualize the entire workflow around assessment. This is done at both the course and program levels. At a course level, assessors are challenged to self-evaluate their current assessment practices and are provided guidance for improvement. All relevant documentation (e.g., assessment matrices, test questions, evaluations) is stored on a course dashboard. At the curriculum level, assessment information is aggregated and visualized through multiple dashboards to provide insight into the alignment between program objectives, course learning objectives, teaching activities, and assessment strategies. The application provides a comprehensive picture of which outcomes are assessed at what level, in what way, and how often. This information serves as valuable input into the PDCA cycle and allows stakeholders to have a productive dialogue and take subsequent actions to sustainably improve assessment quality.

In E-quality, a distinction is made between three stages: design, administration, and the evaluation stage of testing. The start of the assessment cycle is characterized by the *design* of the assessment. Among other things, this involves the development of an assessment matrix that describes which assessment method is applied and how each assessment aligns with the course objectives and program objectives. Furthermore, the application provides the opportunity to upload the assessment items or questions to review them with colleagues. Supporting questions related to the four quality criteria subsequently help the teacher ensure the development of a high-quality assessment. The second stage of the assessment

> **Box 9-1   OVERVIEW AND DESCRIPTION OF THE QUALITY CRITERIA THAT ARE USED IN THE TOOL**
>
> **E-Quality**
>
> **Learning impact:** At all levels (single assessment, course, and curriculum), insight into the impact on learning is provided by the application. For example, at a course level, applied assessment strategies should logically build on each other and align with learning and teaching strategies. At the curriculum level, all applied assessments should be strategically chosen and planned to optimally support and enhance a student's journey toward accomplishing the defined program outcomes.
>
> **Reliability:** The application provides educators support in their thinking about reliability. At the level of a single assessment method, insight is provided into the psychometric properties of the test and guidelines are provided to support standardization of the assessment. At the course and curriculum levels, insight is provided to monitor whether appropriate sampling is applied across different measurement conditions.
>
> **Validity:** The interpretative validity argumentation perspective is applied as an underlying structure to assist in making a coherent analysis of evidence in support of (or against) interpretations of test score meaning. At the assessment method level, the alignment between an assessment method, the course learning objectives, and the program outcomes are visualized. Furthermore, at the curriculum level, insight is provided on how each assessment method in each course contributes to accomplishing the program outcomes.
>
> **Transparency:** Improving assessment quality and changing assessment culture toward one focused on improvement and learning is complex and above all requires a transparent and clear communication about its goals. Modern assessment strategies in competency-based education (e.g., programmatic assessment) are especially new to both students and teachers and require training. The application provides guidance to educators in providing clear and effective communication strategies regarding the applied assessment strategies.

cycle is the *administration* of the test. In this phase, it is especially important to safeguard transparent and effective communication with the students. The application supports this stage by addressing those issues that are relevant. The third stage involves the *evaluation* of the assessment cycle. Besides allowing documentation of results and some psychometric properties of the test, support is given to the teacher with respect to the other quality criteria. For example, based on input from student evaluations, the level of impact of the test on students' learning is explored. When the three stages of the assessment are completed, actions for improvement are formulated to close the PDCA cycle. This is an important feature of the application for continuous and sustainable improvement of assessment quality. By documenting the cycle over several years, a rich and meaningful database is created. Besides allowing teachers to learn from each other, this also allows a smooth transition when responsibilities change between different teachers.

At the curriculum level, a transparent overview of assessment quality is often lacking. E-quality provides a solution for this by visualizing aggregated information at a program level with respect to the program outcomes, assessment methods, assessment metrics, self-evaluation, and assessment documents. Direct insight is provided in potential issues related to constructive alignment, validity, learning impact, reliability, and transparency. Depending on the question or quality at stake, different overviews can be created. This information is essential for teachers, educational directors, examination board members, and accreditation organizations. It would provide direct input to start a meaningful dialogue and discuss relevant actions to increase quality.

Outcomes and Lessons Learned

By aggregating and visualizing relevant information at both course and curriculum levels, the application E-quality aims to foster a dialogue between stakeholders involved in the assessment program. It is essential that the system supports the process of steering toward a quality culture that is focused on learning. As a consequence, it has to be adaptive to future changes and contextual differences in assessment strategies to allow educational programs to sustainably enhance and assure assessment quality.

CONTINUUM OF THEORETICAL PERSPECTIVES ON ASSESSMENT QUALITY

Psychometric Perspective

Because of its strong historical roots, the psychometric perspective is frequently used as a quality indicator for assessments [33,34]. Especially in the early days, it mainly focused on the test score a learner obtained, which was assumed to reflect the intended learner characteristic (e.g., ability level, level of understanding). Because this characteristic is—usually—not assessed directly (e.g., length, weight), it is often coined as a "latent characteristic" (i.e., construct). The main aim of the psychometric perspective is determining whether the test score primarily reflects the latent characteristic (i.e., construct relevance, true score) instead of an unintended characteristic (i.e., construct irrelevance, error score). Measurement error could be the result of systematic errors (e.g., test construction such as unclear item formulation) as well as random errors (e.g., test circumstances such as a noisy test room). Preferably, the measurement error score should be close to zero. To examine the measurement error, the psychometric perspective introduced two quality indicators (i.e., validity and reliability) and associated (mainly statistics-oriented) quality assurance procedures.

Validity

Originally, validity was coined as one concept aimed at verifying whether the assessment actually assesses the intended latent characteristic. Messick [35], for example, operationalized validity into several different conceptualizations, each focusing on a specific validity aspect. Because it is beyond the scope of this chapter to discuss them all, a common simplified distinction will be used here. *Content validity* focuses on whether the assessment covers all relevant aspects of the content domain it intends to measure. If, for example, a relevant aspect is not included or an irrelevant aspect is included, the content validity of the assessment (program) is threatened. A variety of nonstatistical procedures can be utilized at the course and program level to ensure the content validity. For example, domain-specific referencing frames—(inter) national standards, for example—and scientific literature, as well as consultations with domain experts could be appropriate for this purpose. *Construct validity* focuses on the extent to which the assessment's items (e.g., type, number, item formulation, scoring) can capture all relevant aspects properly. If, for example, there is a mismatch between the level of understanding (e.g., insight) and the type of items (e.g., multiple-choice) the construct validity of the assessment (program) is threatened. An example of nonstatistical procedures is the construction and discussion of an overview of relevant aspects and associated mastery levels and items (i.e., assessment matrix). Furthermore, the four-eyes principle (i.e., at least one other colleague is involved in the construction of the assessment) and pilots could be utilized to verify whether the item formulation is clear for the assessees. *Criterion validity* focuses on how closely the results of the assessment correspond to the results of a different assessment. This could be a different assessment aimed at assessing one or more of the same aspects. In case a high correlation between assessment scores is obtained, this provides a good indication that the assessment indeed assesses what it claims. It could also be a different assessment that will take place at a later point in time. In this case, the degree to which the assessment (e.g., average grade year 1) predicts (e.g., regression analysis) the aspect that will be assessed (e.g., score bachelor's thesis) is examined.

Reliability

Whereas validity focuses on which latent characteristic should be assessed, reliability is aimed at verifying how consistently this is done [36,37]. Often a distinction between internal and external reliability is made. *Internal reliability* focuses on the consistency of results across items within a specific assessment. In case the item scores for (a specific aspect of) the assessment point in different directions (e.g., low correlations), this threatens the internal reliability of the assessment. Commonly utilized statistical procedures for examining this are the Cronbach's alpha (i.e., correlating all item scores) and split-half (i.e., correlating item scores between comparable subparts) technique. When, for example, making decisions about individual learners, a cutoff score of 0.80 is often advised [38].

   External reliability focuses on the consistency of results across assessments or assessors. Consistency across assessments refers to the stability of the results over time. In case the same assessment is administered at different moments in time (i.e., test-retest analysis), the assessment score should show high correlations. Otherwise, the external reliability of the assessment is threatened. Consistency across assessors refers to the extent to which assessors give consistent ratings for the assessed latent characteristic. In case the ratings from two assessors for a specific student characteristic (e.g., competency) differ substantially, this raises questions about the external validity. Was the latent characteristic assessed adequately or did some other student characteristic (e.g., personal trait) or improper application of the assessment's scoring rules affect the ratings? To address this, it is advisable to organize so-called calibration sessions in which (potential) differences in scoring or grading are established and discussed in order to come to an agreement about the scoring or grading [1,39]. Although examining the reliability of the whole assessment is valuable, the reader might also be interested in additional perspectives on this matter. Estimations of reliability can be done through three generations of theories: (1) classical test theory, (2) generalizability theory, and (3) item-response theory (e.g., [34,40,41]). These topics fall, however, outside the scope of the current chapter.

Edumetric Perspective

Although the psychological and statistics domains contributed significantly to the development of the psychometric perspective, other perspectives might also be feasible. The rise of other domains (e.g., educational sciences) led to the development of perspectives on quality assurance that go beyond the psychometric characteristics of an assessment (program). In contrast to the psychometric perspective, the edumetric perspective is not focused on the validity or reliability of an assessment but stresses the importance of two other quality indicators [42]. The rationale behind this is that a measurement outcome (e.g., test, program) should be interpreted with a broader perspective in mind instead of focusing solely on the outcome itself [23,24,43]. Assessors quite often use scores for the assessment of learning—namely, making decisions regarding selection and qualification. Because in these high-stake cases the consequences can be severe (e.g., passing or failing a course), it is advisable to raise the bar for the quality assurances (e.g., higher quality demands, re-sit). Assessors could, however, also use assessment scores to foster the assessees' personal development [44,45]. From the viewpoint of assessment for learning, the score provides an indication of one's mastery level and potential aspects for improvement. Based on this indication, feedback aimed at enhancing one's mastery is provided by a teacher or supervisor. Such an assessment is often coined as low stakes because no severe consequences are attached. Taking the stake of the assessment into account is often coined as the *impact* quality indicator. Several procedures could be utilized to ensure that the impact quality indicator is addressed properly. It should be made clear to assessors as well as assessees which assessments will be administered and what the associated—low or high stakes—consequences will be. In case multiple high-stakes assessments are administered, each assessment should have a substantiable weighing. Furthermore, it is advisable that the principle of constructive alignment is utilized; this means that there is a strong alignment between the learning goals, the learning activities, and the assessment. In case, for example, the learning activities (e.g., focus on insight) deviate from the assessment (e.g., focus on replication) or from the learning goals (e.g., application), this threatens the quality of an assessment (program). The edumetric perspective also advocates the use of the *utility* quality indicator—namely, the (administration of the) assessment needs to be transparent and efficient for both assessors and assessees. It should be clear for the assessors as well as the assessees how the (1) assessment will be administered (e.g., requirements, rules for plagiarism or fraud, timing), (2) scoring rules will be applied, and (3) grades will be determined. This information should be clear for all involved stakeholders and made available at the start of a course. Otherwise, this could threaten the utility quality indicator.

Interpretative Validity Argumentation Perspective: Argument-Based Approach and Evidence-Centered Design Approach

In contrast to distinguishing multiple quality assurance indicators, proponents of the interpretative validity approach advocate the utilization of a different perspective. From their viewpoint, several pitfalls are associated with the utilization of especially the psychometric perspective. First, the variety in psychometric concepts raises the question whether the utilization of a specific procedure should be valued more in comparison to other ones. This raises design choices such as, what should be preferred when a construct is not measured in a reliable manner or when the assessment does not meet the edumetric quality assurance demands? Second, because of new insights other assessment types that capture the knowledge, skills, and attitudes more directly have been introduced. These so-called performance assessments require that assessees carry out a task (i.e., giving a presentation, solving a problem) that enables them to exhibit construct relevant behavior. This deviates from assessment types (i.e., knowledge test, questionnaires) used to capture the mastery level in an indirect manner (i.e., latent variable) and often in comparison to other learners. Based on this critique, proponents of the interpretative validity approach argue that the formal—statistical—arguments on their own are insufficient and that informal arguments (i.e., proper lines of reasoning) are needed when developing quality assurances for assessment (programs).

As depicted in Figure 9-1, informal arguments are often coined in terms of Toulmin's model of argumentation [46]. By doing so, the quality assurance indicators and associated procedures are integrated in one approach to validate the assessment (program). In other words, the interpretative validity argument starts with a *ground*, which usually is the data for the specific (performance) assessment (e.g., poor parking, speed limit violation). Based on the ground, a *claim* is made regarding the meaning and implications of the obtained score (e.g., obtaining the driver license). To ensure that the assessment is valid, it is important to explicate underlying *warrants*, making it reasonable to assume that the assessment captures construct-relevant instead of construct-irrelevant characteristics (e.g., sufficient time, reliable scoring). For a sound argumentation, the warrants have to be substantiated with *backings*—namely, theoretical (e.g., certification board) as well as empirical (e.g., time measured, interrater reliability) evidence. Based on the provided grounds, claims, warrants, and backings, the quality of the interpretative argument can be determined in terms of the *qualifier* (i.e., low, medium, or high). Although there are hardly any guidelines for this, a higher quality is required in case the stakes associated with the assessment are higher. As common in theories about argumentation, it is also valuable to verify whether *rebuttals* (i.e., counterarguments),

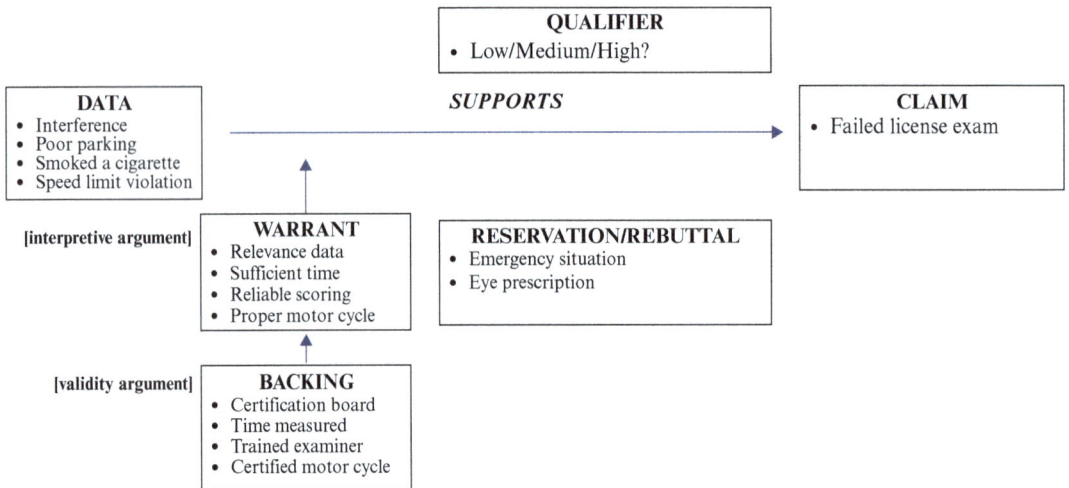

Figure 9-1 • Example of interpretative validity argumentation: motor cycle driver license.

that undermine the quality of reasoning or provide an indication of construct irrelevance could be provided.

Two frequently mentioned interpretative validity approaches are the argument-based approach [29] and evidence-centered design (ECD) approach [30]. The *argument-based approach* advocates that the performance and associated decision are interrelated properly (top-down or bottom-up); that is, a program should ensure that the assessment performance (e.g., answers to an exam) is scored properly (e.g., scoring or grading rules) and can be generalized to the test domain (e.g., suitability assessment conditions). Furthermore, the content of the assessment should properly reflect the course as well as the educational program's learning outcomes (i.e., extrapolation) and are a proper indication of a student's performance in practice (i.e., interpretation). To do so, all four types of inferences—scoring, generalization, extrapolation, and interpretation—have to be substantiated with informal arguments. This means that for each type of inference, at least one claim and associated warrants and backings (theoretical and empirical) have to be drawn up (see Figure 9-2, left side).

The *ECD approach* advocates that assessment (programs) should be developed in a top-down and stepwise manner (see Figure 9-2, right side). The *domain analysis layer* starts with analyzing the (sub)domain for which the assessments will be developed. This should result in a general description of the types of knowledge, skills, and attributes (KSAs) that need to be assessed. In the *domain modeling layer*, an informal argument has to

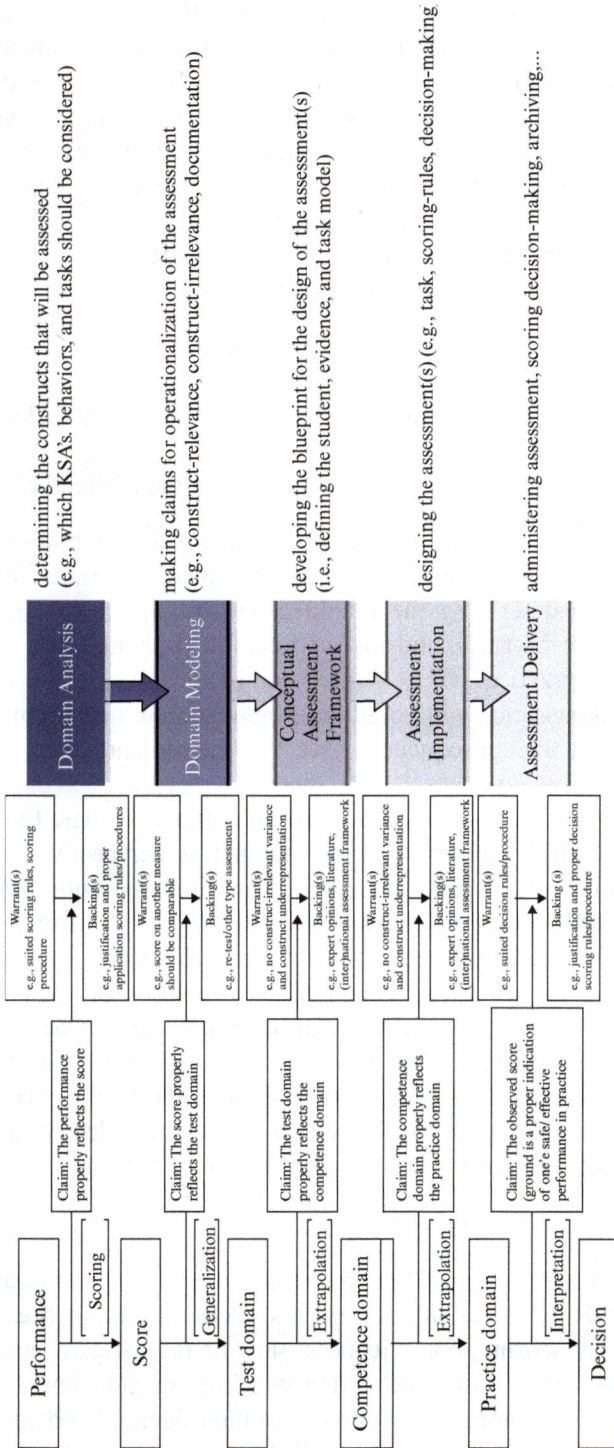

Figure 9-2 • Overview argument-based (left) and evidence–centered design (right) approach.

be drawn up to operationalize the assessment of the selected KSAs, which means that the goal (i.e., claim) of the assessment and assessment design decisions (i.e., warrants) have to be formulated. In addition, indications of theoretical and empirical evidence (i.e., backings) and potential rebuttals (i.e., indications of construct irrelevance) have to be provided. In the *conceptual assessment framework*, a blueprint (i.e., concrete design guidelines) for the actual design of the assessments will be developed based on the informal argument. The blueprint defines the design specification for three different aspect (i.e., models), namely, the:

1. student model and guidelines for operationalizing KSA's into performance behavior,
2. task model and guidelines for developing assessment tasks that can elicit the behavior, and
3. evidence model and guidelines for scoring the elicited behavior.

In the *assessment implementation layer*, the design guidelines will be utilized to develop assessments and all related materials. For example, documents describing the intended performance behavior, assessment tasks, scoring rules, and instructions for applying these materials to educational practices will be written and handed over to the assessors. Thereafter, assessments will be administered, scored, and archived, and decisions about the consequences have to be made and acted on in the *assessment delivery layer*.

When drawing up the claims, warrants, and backings, the aspects addressed by the psychometric and edumetric perspective are often integrated into the informal argument. The discussed approaches (i.e., argument-based and evidence-centered design) both utilize a holistic construct-centered design approach in which at least one informal argument should be drawn up. There are also two main differences between both approaches. First, whereas the argument-based approach requires an informal argument for each inference, only one argument is drawn up in the evidence-centered approach (i.e., domain modeling). Second, the evidence-centered approach addresses the assessment delivery and implementation, but the argument-based approach does not.

Reflection on the Perspectives

Assessment is a challenging endeavor at both the course and educational program levels [21,45,47,48]. It involves decision-making (i.e., design, administration, scoring, consequences—low or high stakes—and acting on the consequences) for which often no clear-cut guidelines are readily available. Decision-making thus places high demands on the professional judgment of the responsible stakeholders (e.g., teachers, program directors, examination boards). From a theoretical perspective, this section has been aimed at offering some rules of thumb (i.e., quality indicators) and associated quality assurance procedures. As indicated, solely utilizing the psychometric perspective (i.e., validity, reliability) or an edumetric perspective (i.e., utility, impact) could jeopardize the quality of the assessment (program). To this end, it is advisable to take both perspectives into account in the decision-making process [2]. One approach would be to draw up separate descriptions for all four quality indicators in which quality assurances descriptions, procedures, and safeguards are clearly defined. Another approach would be to utilize a more integrative perspective such as the interpretative validity argumentation approach [29,30]. Although often utilized for standardized—high-stake—tests, this approach might offer valuable insights for the decision-making process for other types of assessment and assessment programs. In other words, clearly stating the goal (i.e., claim), the assumption (i.e., warrants), and the theoretical and empirical evidence (i.e., backings) provides more insight into the line of reasoning behind the assessment (program). Whereas the interpretative validity argumentation perspective might require a higher investment (e.g., resources, conceptualization, fine-tuning), it can support decision-makers in explicating their—often implicit—arguments about the assessment programs to each other and other stakeholders. By doing so, the line of reasoning underlying the assessment program becomes more transparent and might serve as input for discussions aimed at enhancing its quality.

▌CONCLUSION

Having a sound assessment program is vital for both internal and external stakeholders. It requires a systematic approach to assessment and learning that incorporates learning and assessment practices that are complementary to each other and embedded throughout a program of study [14,17]. The assurance of such a program serves purposes of both accountability and improvement. In this chapter we discussed practical guidelines and theoretical perspectives that refer to the quality of an assessment program. High-quality standards (i.e., psychometric and edumetric criteria) and related procedures and plans (i.e., input, process, output) should be integrated in systems of internal and external quality assurance. This implies establishing a continuous and iterative process of monitoring, analysis and action to regularly review and renew the assessment program.

In this chapter two worked out examples are provided to give insight in how this can be practiced. To ensure continuous improvement and feed the possibility of a quality-assured curriculum, we need more than written documents and plans. The case studies show us the roles and responsibilities that internal and external stakeholders should have in this process. To be able to reflect on current actions and formulate new goals, the line of reasoning underlying the assessment program should be transparent and insight is needed into what the underlying quality indicators and procedures are. This also could serve as input for discussion and dialogue between different stakeholders about the organization's ambition regarding assessment, the current state of assessment quality, and about realistic short- and long-term measures to improve assessment quality. Steering toward a quality culture that is focused on learning enables programs to sustainably enhance and assure the assessment quality. However, this can be a laborious and difficult process. Box 9-2 lists some suggestions for avoiding common pitfalls in this process.

Box 9-2 AVOIDING COMMON PITFALLS IN QUALITY ASSURANCE OF AN ASSESSMENT PROGRAM

Avoiding Common Pitfalls

- Teachers often have considerable autonomy in developing assessment procedures within their courses. On the one hand, this is desirable because they are the experts in their own fields. On the other hand, courses may risk becoming too self-contained, resulting in an unaligned curriculum in which learning processes are not structurally embedded and monitored. To avoid fragmentation of the curriculum into unrelated subjects and assessments and to enhance constructive alignment, consultation between teachers should be facilitated. Moreover, the rationale of how the curriculum is structured and how each course contributes to this structure should be familiar to and discussed among teachers.
- Writing policy plans and other assessment documents that give a profound insight into the content and structure of the assessment program can take a significant amount of time. Often these documents are used for accountability purposes and only composed when programs face an accreditation. Consequently, these documents reflect a "paper reality" that is not recognized by practice. Avoid these "paper realities" by incorporating the documentation and discussion on assessment within daily quality assurances polices and use it as a mean to sustainably improve the assessment quality.
- Often, the preparation for accreditation is experienced as stimulating, but it also can be quite a heavy burden. For many educational the assurance of assessment quality is a (major) topic when facing an accreditation. Reduce the workload for accreditation activities by structurally and continuously embedding assessment quality in structural quality assurance procedures—for example, by utilizing assessment quality assurance procedures according to the PDCA cycle at both the course and the program levels.

REFERENCES

1. Bloxham S, Price M. External Examining: Fit for Purpose? *Stud High Educ.* 2013;1(13):1–17.

2. Gerritsen-van Leeuwenkamp KJ, Joosten-ten Brinke D, Kester L. Assessment Quality in Tertiary Education: An Integrative Literature Review. *Stud Educ Eval.* 2017;55:94–116.

3. Secolsky C, Denison D, eds. *Handbook on Measurement, Assessment, and Evaluation in Higher Education.* New York: Taylor & Francis; 2017.

4. Baartman L, Gulikers J, Dijkstra A. Factors Influencing Assessment Quality in Higher Vocational Education. *Assessment & Evaluation in Higher Education.* 2013;38(8):1–20. doi:10.1080/02602938.2013.771133

5. Maassen NAM, Hopster-den Otter D, Wools S, et al. Quality of Assessments Within Reach: Review Study of Research and Results of the Quality of Assessments. *Pedagog Stud.* 2015;92(6):380–393.

6. Baartman L, Kloppenburg R, Prins F. Kwaliteit van toetsprogramma's. In: *Toetsen in Het Hoger Onderwijs.* Houten, The Netherlands: Bohn Stafleu van Loghum. 2017:37–49.

7. Van der Vleuten CPM, Schuwirth LWT, Driessen EW, et al. A Model for Programmatic Assessment Fit for Purpose. *Med Teach.* 2012;34(3):205–214.

8. Sluijsmans D, Joosten-ten Brinke D, van Schilt-Mol T. *Kwaliteit van toetsing onder de loep. Handvatten om de kwaliteit van toetsing in het Hoger Onderwijs te analyseren, verbeteren en borgen.* 2nd ed. Antwerpen-Apeldoorn: Garant; 2015.

9. Jensen HT, Aspelin M, Devinsky F, et al. *Quality Culture in European universities: A Bottom-Up Approach Report on the Three Rounds of the Quality Culture Project 2002–2006.* Brussels: European University Association; 2006.

10. Hobson R, Rolland S, Rotgans J, et al. Quality Assurance, Benchmarking, Assessment and Mutual International Recognition of Qualifications. *Eur J Dent Educ.* 2008;12(Suppl.1):92–100.

11. Tam M. Outcomes-Based Approach to Quality Assessment and Curriculum Improvement in Higher Education. *Qual Assur Educ.* 2014;22(2):158–168.

12. Dijkstra J, Galbraith R, Hodges BD, et al. Expert Validation of Fit-for-Purpose Guidelines for Designing Programmes of Assessment. *BMC Med Educ.* 2012; 12(1):12–20.

13. Biggs J, Tang C. *Teaching for Quality Learning at University: What the Student Does.* McGraw-Hill Education. UK; 2011.

14. Norcini J, Anderson MB, Bollela V, et al. Consensus Framework for Good Assessment. *Med Teach.* 2018;40(11):1102–1109.

15. Gagné RM. Learning Outcomes and Their Effects: Useful Categories of Human Performance. *Am Psychol.* 1984;39(4):377–385.

16. NVAO Nederlands-Vlaamse Accreditatie Organisatie. Assessment and Demonstration of Achieved Learning Outcomes: Recommendations and Good Practices. http://ecahe.eu/assets/uploads/2018/01/Report-Achieved-Learning-Outcomes-Recommendations-and-Good-Practices-2016.pdf

17. Boud D, Associates. *Assessment 2020. Seven Propositions for Assessment Reform in Higher Education.* Sydney: Australian Learning and Teaching Council; 2010.

18. Frank JR, Danoff D. The CanMEDS Initiative: Implementing an Outcomes-Based Framework of Physician Competencies. *Med Teach*. 2007;29(7):642–647.
19. Bok HGJ, Jaarsma DADC, Teunissen PW, van der Vleuten CPM, van Beukelen P. Development and Validation of a Competency Framework for Veterinarians. *J Vet Med Educ*. 2011;38(3):262–269.
20. Dill D. *Quality Assurance in Higher Education: Practices and Issues*. University of North Carolina; 2007.
21. Baartman LKJ, Bastiaens TJ, Kirschner PA, van der Vleuten PM. Evaluating Assessment Quality in Competence-Based Education: A Qualitative Comparison of Two Frameworks. *Educ Res Rev*. 2007;2:114–129.
22. Baartman LKJ, Prins FJ, Kirschner PA, van der Vleuten PM. Self-Evaluation of Assessment Programs: A Cross-Case Analysis. *Eval Program Plann*. 2011; 34(3):206–216.
23. Baartman LKJ, Prins FJ, Kirschner PA, van der Vleuten CPM. Determining the Quality of Competence Assessment Programs: A Self-Evaluation Procedure. *Stud Educ Eval*. 2007;33(3-4):258–281.
24. Baartman LKJ, Bastiaens TJ, Kirschner PA, Van der Vleuten CPM. Teachers' Opinions on Quality Criteria for Competency Assessment Programs. *Teach Teach Educ*. 2007;23(6):857–867.
25. Segers M, Dochy F. Quality Assurance in Higher Education: Theoretical Considerations and Empirical Evidence. *Stud Educ Eval*. 1996;22(2):115–137.
26. Gibbs G, Dunbar-Goddet H. Characterising Programme-Level Assessment Environments That Support Learning. *Assess Eval High Educ*. 2009;34(4): 481–489.
27. Van der Vleuten CPM. Revisiting Assessing Professional Competence: From Methods to Programmes. *Med Educ*. 2016;50(9):885–888.
28. Grant D, Mergen E, Widrick S. Quality Management in US Higher Education. *Total Qual Manag*. 2002;13(2):207–215.
29. Kane M. Certification Testing as an Illustration of Argument-Based Validation. *Meas Interdiscip Res Perspect*. 2004;2(3):135–170.
30. Mislevy RJ, Haertel GD. Implications of Evidence-Centered Design for Educational Assessment. *Educ Meas Issues Pract*. 2006;25(4):6–20.
31. Thijs A, van den Akker J. *Leerplan in Ontwikkeling [Curricula in Development*. Enschede: SLO; 2009.
32. Valcke M. *Onderwijskunde Als Ontwerpwetenschap: Deel 1 En 2. Educational Sciences as a Design Discipline: Part 1 and 2*. EAN: 97894. ACCO Publisher; 2018.
33. Schoenherr JR, Hamstra SJ. Psychometrics and its discontents: an historical perspective on the discourse of the measurement tradition. *Adv Heal Sci Educ*. 2016;21(3):719–729.
34. Traub R. Classical Test Theory in Historical Perspective. *Educ Meas Issues Pract*. 1997;16:8–14.
35. Messick S. Standards of Validity and the Validity of Standards in Performance Asessment. *Educ Meas Issues Pract*. 2005;14(4):5–8.

36. Feldt LS, Brennan RL. Reliability. In: Linn L, ed. *Educational Measurement*. 3rd ed. New York: American Council on Education/Macmillan; 1989:105–146.

37. Moss PA. The Meaning and Consequences of "Reliability." *J Educ Behav Stat*. 2004;29(2):245–249.

38. Cho E, Kim S. Cronbach's Coefficient Alpha: Well Known but Poorly Understood. *Organ Res Methods*. 2015;18:207–230.

39. O'Connell B, de Lange P, Freeman M, et al. Does Calibration Reduce Variability in the Assessment of Accounting Learning Outcomes? *Assess Eval High Educ*. 2016;41(3):331–349.

40. Brennan RL. Generalizability Theory. *Educ Meas Issues Pract*. 1992;11(4):27–34.

41. Sijtsma K, Molenaar I. *Introduction to Nonparametric Item Response Theory*. Thousand Oaks, CA: Sage; 2002.

42. Carver RP. Two Dimensions of Tests: Psychometric and Edumetric. *Am Psych*. 1974;29(7):512–518.

43. Poldner E, Simons PRJ, Wijngaards G, van der Schaaf MF. Quantitative Content Analysis Procedures to Analyse Students' Reflective Essays: A Methodological Review of Psychometric and Edumetric Aspects. *Educ Res Rev*. 2012;7(1):19–37.

44. Black P, Wiliam D. Classroom Assessment and Pedagogy. *Assess Educ Princ Policy Pract*. 2018;25(6):551–575.

45. Heitink MC, van der Kleij FM, Veldkamp BP, Schildkamp K, Kippers WB. A Systematic Review of Prerequisites for Implementing Assessment for Learning in Classroom Practice. *Educ Res Rev*. 2016;17:50–62.

46. Toulmin S, Rieke R, Janik A. *An Introduction to Reasoning*. New York: Macmillan; 1979.

47. Pellegrino JW, Dibello LV, Goldman SR. A Framework for Conceptualizing and Evaluating the Validity of Instructionally Relevant Assessments. *Educ Psychol*. 2016;51(1).

48. Sadler DR. The Futility of Attempting to Codify Academic Achievement Standards. *High Educ*. 2014;67(3):273–288.

10 Quality Assurance of Assessment During Major Disruptions

Richard B. Hays, Bunmi S. Malau-Aduli, Tim J. Wilkinson, and Cees P.M. van der Vleuten

CHAPTER HIGHLIGHTS

- The COVID-19 pandemic has initiated rapid fundamental changes to the delivery of assessment in medical education and this emphasizes the need for a holistic programmatic approach to assessment to ensure quality and foster continuous improvement.
- This chapter focuses on future assessment developments and the acceleration resulting from the pandemic.
- It also highlights the impact on teaching and learning and how this is an opportunity to develop better learning and assessment methods.
- The impact on accreditation processes and how technology will shape these responses are also considered.

▌ORIENTATION TO THE CHAPTER

In this book, we have presented discussions of the latest thinking on a range of issues that are relevant to the quality assurance (QA) of assessment in medical education and most likely across all health professions education programs. The timing was interesting because the book was commissioned just before the COVID-19 pandemic, and most chapters were written during the first wave of the pandemic. Chapters cover the rationale for assessment QA, the roles and responsibilities of QA assessors, assessment of knowledge and clinical competence, Work Based Assessment (WBA), programmatic assessment, use of technology, and standardization. The publisher challenged us with the question, How meaningful are these topics in an era of major disruption to "normal business"? Therefore, this final chapter draws together elements of these discussions in the context of the changes forced by the major disruption experienced by all. Are there lessons to be learned from these experiences? We address the question, to what degree will the disruption lead to longer-term changes to assessment practices and how they are quality assured? We begin with the recent pandemic as a case study (**Case 10-1**) and then present comments on the international impact and responses.

Case 10-1: A Major Disruption

During December 2019, a series of cases with an unusual acute respiratory system disease were identified in one region of the People's Republic of China. This disease appeared to spread rapidly and to have high complication and mortality rates. By early January 2020, it became clear that there was an outbreak of a potentially new infectious disease, a coronavirus that may have mutated and "jumped" species from other animals to humans. Initially, this was thought to be a problem for this one region of one country, and the world watched while that region went into "lockdown" and reoriented health care toward strict public health measures and expanding acute critical care resources. Health professionals were also getting ill and dying. Medical education almost ceased, and both teaching faculty and more senior students were drawn into providing clinical services. Travel restrictions were imposed within that region and between that region and other parts of the world, but by mid- to late February it was clear that the infection had already spread well beyond the initial region, particularly to international destinations with strong business, family, and therefore travel links to China. One by one, other nations reported rapid increases in the numbers of people both with the disease and dying of the acute respiratory syndrome. These nations responded, mostly too late to prevent a first wave epidemic, with substantial changes to health care and varying degrees of society lockdown, in which medical education could not continue. Again, teaching clinicians and senior students became integral components of the workforce. Nonurgent care was postponed for several weeks, even months. The focus was on increasing emergency department and intensive care unit beds, equipment, and staffing. Even where students could attend, they were exposed to both risks and a skewed clinical case mix that did not necessarily match the breadth of learning objectives. Assessment was similarly affected because written assessment had to move to online methods; clinical assessments such as Objective Structured Clinical Examinations (OSCEs) and WBAs were not possible. For the medical education programs in the Northern Hemisphere, end-of-year and pregraduation progress decisions had to be either deferred or based on previous assessments. Although the severity of the first wave, its impact, and the responses varied between countries, this massive global disruption affected almost all aspects of human existence. How long this disruption will last, and how far ahead is another similar major disruption, are common topics of discussion.

INTRODUCTION—GETTING BACK TO "NORMAL" BUSINESS

One of the greatest challenges in writing this chapter is that we do not know when or if life will return to normal. The pandemic has disrupted almost every facet of life on which medical education depends. Preventing new waves of the pandemic requires achieving herd immunity, ideally through an effective vaccine that is administered globally. At the time of writing, in mid-2021 the global vaccination rollout is underway, but not before second and third waves occurred in some countries. Significant disruptions are likely to continue for some time. The "new normal" may be a fluctuation between relative freedom and degrees of restrictions to manage further waves until "natural" herd immunity develops. Along that path are continued major disruptions and potentially many more deaths. Further, the possibility must be considered that another global disruption may emerge, possibly further pandemics, global conflicts, or something like a substantial meteor or asteroid collision. Other less global disruptions may be more likely such as earthquakes, severe storms, drought, and so on, which are more localized and allow faster recovery. A technological failure such as an Internet breakdown could cause a different type of disruption. These events require us to "think on our feet," innovate while we continue to deliver services, and think about problems in new ways. Such tensions often provide the opportunity to develop previously unconsidered solutions. But we need principles to follow so that we can have a framework to try to predict and evaluate the effects.

The new normal, called by some a *return to better*, may be a continuation of some current strategies and a state of constant readiness to adapt should a further disruption recur. Are there lessons to be drawn from this recent experience for application in future disruptions from any cause?

We propose the conceptual model presented in Figure 10-1 to explain the relationship between medical education and the surrounding influences. The center of the model is the focus of this chapter: medical education. This diagram is not to suggest that medical education is the central issue during the pandemic, but rather a way of looking at medical education through the surrounding influences that determine almost everything that happens within medical education.

In addition, face-to-face education methods have been affected and online methods have been adopted more broadly at all levels of education.

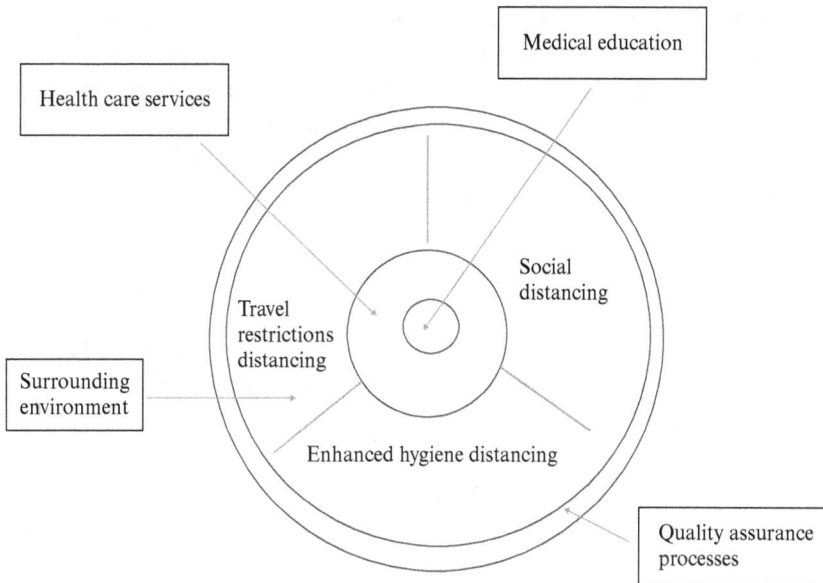

Figure 10-1 • A conceptual model for the interaction of surrounding influences on health professional education.

The second layer is health care in which medical education is embedded firmly. During the pandemic, the whole health-care system has been reoriented to focus on two specialties—public health and critical care. Elective surgery, chronic disease management, and the management of almost every other non–COVID-19 illness have been deferred. Travel restrictions mean that both patients and clinicians cannot get to health-care facilities for nonurgent care. Clinical placements have been canceled, particularly for more junior students. For more senior students and postgraduate trainees, clinical placements have continued, but the case mix has been distorted to reflect the critical care focus, potentially placing limits on breadth of learning and progress through undergraduate and postgraduate curricula.

The third layer includes public health strategies that affect the way that civilization works and appear to have been effective in limiting the effects of the pandemic. These include enhanced hygiene measures, social distancing, and travel restrictions. All these strategies have influenced ways of working in almost every sector of society, including health care and medical education services. Quality assurance processes are placed in the outer layer because they focus on the inner two layers but must function through the surrounding influences. For example, visits by QA teams to observe teaching, learning, and assessment and to discuss faculty and student support are currently being conducted via video-conferencing as well as conferences that require travel. How these issues interact and affect assessment in medical education is difficult to predict and will be of great interest in the coming months and years.

▍MAINTAINING ENHANCED HYGIENE PRACTICES

Medical professionals may understand this issue better than most because they already wash their hands frequently. Will this continue to be applied on a much broader scale for everyone entering and leaving workplaces and education facilities? Until vaccination has slowed the spread of the coronavirus, elbow coughing makes sense and should continue, just as handshaking, hugging, and air-kissing may disappear. Huddles over a coffee may be discouraged. Social gatherings may look quite different or be reduced. Absences from work of students and staff while even mildly ill will be the norm, and the disruptions this may cause will have to be managed. The concept of attendance may have to evolve. Although nonclinical assessment may have little impact on hygiene and be managed by online examination methods, clinical assessment is much more difficult to adapt because candidates are often required to conduct clinical procedures such as physical examination on several patients within a short period of time. Should personal protective equipment be worn by patients, candidates, and assessors during clinical assessments? There are reports of OSCEs that include additional hygiene measures [1], but OSCEs are still logistically complex events that mix together people from many places. Further, do the risks of disease transmission increase when students are assessed on real patient encounters in the workplace?

▍MAINTAINING SOCIAL DISTANCING PRACTICES

If a word cloud were to be created from press releases during 2020, the term *social distancing* might come in second to *unprecedented*. Although relatively new, the concept permeates almost every strategy used to delay the spread of COVID-19 and affects every aspect of human existence. However, what will this look like as lockdowns ease? Travel between home, education facilities, and health-care facilities may remain more difficult because most forms of transport require people to be extremely close to each other. Workspaces have recently embraced open-plan designs and "hot desks." Lecture halls and tutorial rooms are designed to allow about 1 square meter per occupant, not the 4 square meters recommended to limit droplet infection spread. Recreational spaces are designed similarly to be more crowded than guidelines allow. The impact of social interaction on working and learning may not be well understood. Some but not all workers are able to work from home. Some but not all learning and assessment can be achieved by remote methods. Activities that require thinking or talking can often be undertaken just as easily remotely, including through videoconferencing. Activities that require touching such as physical examination pose greater challenges. Perhaps most importantly, the situations where our learners witness and participate in team interactions may be harder to capture. How does a clinical team prioritize which patient to see first? How does the senior doctor know that the person in one room was sicker than a similar person in another? These judgments are hard to describe and hard to teach, but sometimes can be picked up by learners—provided they are physically colocated with other health workers.

Written assessment can be delivered online, although proctoring is less robust. Conducting clinical assessment is much more challenging because distances between patients, candidates, and assessors is usually less than recommended social distancing practices. Is it possible to "spread" an OSCE over a much greater physical space, or will station numbers have to be reduced, which is likely to threaten validity and reliability? Could risks be minimized by remote monitoring of candidate–patient interactions and using simulated patients as the assessors, as is currently used in large OSCE test centers such as those used by the National Board of Medical Education, the Australian Medical Council, and the Royal College of General Practitioners? Alternatively, have OSCEs become too risky to contemplate because of their mixing of candidates, patients (real or simulated), and examiners from many places into a single location? One model to contemplate is that adopted by the Australian College of Rural and Remote Medicine, where a portfolio of assessments includes a "remote" multistation clinical examination in which examiners move rooms electronically to observe candidates [2,3]. This appears to work well, although applying it on a large scale may be difficult.

▎ CONTINUED TRAVEL RESTRICTIONS

Awareness of the spread of highly infectious diseases is delayed by incubation periods and periods of early prodromal symptoms. During the current pandemic, outbreaks were often not noticed for as many as up to 2 weeks after contact. This has major implications for health care and medical education because students and staff often visit hospitals, community clinics, and nursing care homes within a relatively brief time span. During the pandemic, strict restrictions were applied to travel between clinical facilities and to and from home. A continuation of these restrictions on mobility between health-care facilities may have continuing implications for learning and assessment, limiting integration of health care, learning, and assessment. Should there be quarantine periods between placements at different sites? Should clinical assessment be restricted to patients, learners, and assessors who normally work together? This has been reported as an OSCE adaptation at one site [1]. How does this affect the breadth of the base (validity) of an assessment judgment? How does being assessed only by examiners who know the candidates affect the potential for bias?

Another aspect of travel restriction is the impact on travel further afield, which may limit the use of external examiners and other forms of international interaction around assessment theories and practices such as sabbaticals and conferences. The value of conferences may be underestimated, perhaps because their greatest contribution to advances in academic development is what happens around formal presentations in corridors, breaks, and social events. All participants benefit from developing and expanding personal networks, the most likely source of learning about and sharing experiences in assessment practices. Many research projects and publications have been seeded by intense discussions in the same time zone with people who have similar interests but different levels of experience and expertise. Addressing this potential gap in academic development may require some innovation beyond the webinar technology that is now ubiquitous.

IMPACT ON CLINICAL LEARNING AND ASSESSMENT

Although the impact of the pandemic on clinical case mix has been variable, depending on the severity of the pandemic in different locations, as a rule clinical engagement for more junior students has been suspended for varying periods—from weeks to several months. Final academic year assessments may have been affected the most, because these assessments require high-stakes decision that certifies readiness to enter the workforce with increased responsibility and less supervision. This meant that assessment could not be delayed until after the pandemic. Indeed, in some cases the decisions were brought forward so that new graduates could enter the workforce sooner. Anecdotally, common strategies appear to be relying more on the judgments of senior faculty in-training ratings and modified, smaller-scale clinical observation assessment. In such cases, it may be even more important to follow explicitly principles of good decision-making, guarding against *groupthink* or group bias and ensuring the collation of a robust body of evidence before making high-stakes decisions.

Strategies to compensate for reduced and limited breadth of real patient exposure have included increasing simulation. *Simulation* is a broad term that ranges from low to high fidelity, and simulation involving technology and mannequins that can adapt or respond to learner decisions appears able to augment authentic clinical learning. However, questions remain about potential limitations to exposure to variations in presentation and management if it were the sole source of clinical exposure [4]. There may now be a drive to develop more and a wider range of high-fidelity simulation cases to broaden the simulation experience, with the products suitable for both learning and assessment, although this is a step away from authenticity. OSCEs often rely on simulated patients, but they have been criticized for assessing only components of health care in nonauthentic settings. In response, WBA has emerged as a stronger approach to assessment, and this trend is increasing. However, almost by definition, WBA cannot include less common or less safe situations where simulation has an important role. Mini-clinical examinations (mini-CEX) and direct observation of procedural skills may be more difficult to implement in sufficient numbers. Case-based discussions and rating scales are still possible, although perhaps based on the narrower clinical case mix. Learning portfolios may provide less information from a narrower range of sources, placing emphasis on the question [5]: How much information from what sources is enough? New methods for documenting learning may be required for more dispersed clinical learning opportunities. There are implications for programmatic assessment, which requires judgments on a larger number of assessment *data points* [6]. Research is needed to address such questions.

▌ TIMING

Should the world recover quickly from the pandemic and further waves do not occur, then health care may well be back to "normal" by the time this book becomes available. This means that the restricted clinical placement duration and clinical case mix exposure experienced by students in 2020 may be limited to those students only. This, of course, is not just a single academic year cohort because clinical engagement has been reduced or altered for every class. For the earlier years, catch-up clinical enrichment may be less challenging because the proportion of clinical engagement in most curricula is smaller. The most affected academic cohort may be the penultimate year cohort, which may have endured severely constrained clinical engagement in parts of the final two years.

On the other hand, some disruption and adaptation may continue for some time. This may mean less integrated and longer blocks in some clinical specialties, contact with only one team at each site, less mobility between sites, and assessment by only the local faculty. Small outbreaks or other less major disruptions may require sudden suspension at one site, quarantine periods, and then a switch to online and simulation-based learning and assessment. Teaching and professional staff may need additional training to enable this.

WHAT ABOUT THE NEXT TIME?

An important question is, What have we learned from this stunning disruption? Even if the whole world is vaccinated and COVID-19 becomes simply part of the routine vaccination schedule, how soon will another pandemic occur? If not a pandemic, then how soon will there be another major disruption? The last pandemic was 100 years ago, when millions died around the world and a vaccine was not possible. Arguably, the last major global disruption was 80 years ago during World War 2—when millions died, economies shrank, and medical education was severely disrupted, with small classes and compression of medical course to produce a much needed workforce. However, we should not assume that the next disruption will be another 80 to 100 years. The new normal should include plans to respond more quickly to any disruption to clinical and education services, building on what has worked during the current disruption. Simply returning to previous assessment practices may represent a "waste" of the effort invested in adapting and developing innovative approaches. The challenge is to continue using innovations that both improve assessment utility as part of a systematic approach to assessment and build resilience to manage future disruptions.

IMPACT ON QUALITY ASSURANCE PROCESSES

Quality assurance may become even more important as the future unfolds. Program delivery may maintain some of the changes in order to be less prone to disruptions. The balance of face-to-face and online methods is likely to change, and the focus on workforce immersion may have to move to more senior students to conserve that valuable resource. Simulation is likely to develop further, most likely virtually, with students learning from banks of more open-ended clinical cases and higher-fidelity responsive simulation models, all of which are accessible through remote technology. Internal QA processes will have to accommodate such changes in the education business model. If more is done online, will there be more errors of examiner judgment and progress decisions because of the more limited data available? Further work is necessary to develop standards and protocols for assessment practices for these different circumstances, and assessors may need different training to follow those new protocols. External expertise can still be brought in, but by remote means, which may potentially limit its utility. The viability of the external examiner model may be open to questions because it may be difficult, for security and confidentiality reasons, to livestream clinical assessment, particularly in the workplace to an external examiner at another site.

External QA processes may face both further constraints and opportunities. Visits may be more difficult, perhaps even unachievable, if social distancing, mobility, and travel restrictions continue. The inclusion in QA teams of *external* members to provide an *outside* perspective may be more difficult; achieving this *presence* is currently being tried through webinar technology. Teams often move between airports, hospitals, community clinics, and so on within a short period of time, potentially posing risks of contamination if any infectious disease is present or about to become evident at any of those sites. Webinar technology can provide for meetings with leaders, teachers, researchers, clinicians, employers, working committees, and students, adding discussion to potentially triangulate the content of written submissions. Observation of teaching and assessment may be possible using livestreaming, but the same concerns exist for external examiners as for any observation of clinical assessment. A possible opportunity is that a wider range of expertise, sometimes quite distant, could be brought by webinar into some discussions. Overall, the impact on discussion may be substantial because QA teams usually collaborate in highly interactive meetings to prepare their reports. This activity may be difficult to achieve to the same degree using technology. Further, as with discussions at conferences, there appears to be value in "being there"—interpersonal chemistry, discussion and inquiry, mismatches between written and observed practice—in forming and communicating judgments that are fair, valid, reliable, and able to inspire quality improvement. There may be an opportunity to develop a new accreditation process that includes remote methods where appropriate and limiting face-to-face methods to a short period of time for a small team to observe specific activities.

▌TECHNOLOGY

Technology is the final heading, because this may be the area of greatest development. The presence of substantial technology and infrastructure in some nations allowed for relatively rapid change from face-to-face to online delivery of education services. However, not all nations have the capability to incorporate technology. Even within wealthier nations, some populations have relatively poor internet access, such as poorer and more remote populations. Furthermore, even where the technology is available, there is need for improvement in the skills of users as well as both hardware and software.

As foreshadowed in the introduction to this chapter, even as this book was being written, the global disruption caused by the COVID-19 pandemic has driven a rapid uptake of technology in both teaching and assessment. The early adaptation of programs to online delivery supported remote learning but demonstrated the need to redesign them to build on the strengths that mixed-mode learning offers. The crisis has also enhanced the role of telemedicine. This practice of *remote* disease management may continue to grow even after COVID is contained, transforming medical care for the long term [7], providing an opportunity to redesign clinical software to either include documentation of related learning or export data to learning management systems. In medical education, an overloaded health-care system prioritized clinical service over learning, with many faculty members and postgraduate learners preoccupied with clinical service commitments. Furthermore, the clinical case mix has been skewed toward emergency care, limiting breadth of exposure to the curriculum. The impact may be greatest on assessment practices, particularly at major decision points such as graduation because traditional assessment methods were not designed for remote delivery.

Case 10-2 is an example of relying on current technology to deliver assessment practices not necessarily designed for online delivery and on a larger scale than normal. Unexpected faults in technology are not uncommon and take time to be corrected, even with the best support. The potential for differences in experience and therefore potential lack of fairness for individual candidates is high. Candidate error is currently unlikely because we are in an era of digital natives (Generations Y and Z), who use technology in day-to-day activities and have unique communication and learning styles, preferring learning through peer collaboration, information sharing, online games, and tests [8]. For educators, who may not be as technology savvy, the challenge is to design teaching and assessment methods that engage and meet the expectations of these digital natives [9]. This includes rapid, effective, and personalized student feedback that

> ### Case 10-2: Unexpected Technology Faults in a National Specialty Certification Examination
>
> The final examination for recognition as a specialist general practitioner in Australia is usually held twice each year. In 2020, the first exam was canceled because parts of the country were in lockdown during the first wave of the pandemic, and plans were made to run both the written and clinical examinations only once and for twice the usual number of candidates using online methods. The written examination was a 3-hour Multiple Choice Question (MCQ) test, and existing software and national broadband access made this feasible. However, on the day of the examination, most candidates could not log in to the examination portal, causing enormous confusion, anxiety, and potential disruption of workforce development. The source of error was not identified, with *congestion*—a common challenge during the pandemic—offered as the most likely problem. The examination was delivered successfully a few weeks later by pen and paper with distributed local invigilation because confidence in technology fell sharply. The OSCE was converted to a videoconferenced series of live "stations" where patient scenarios were discussed over several days to minimize potential disruption. Although successfully implemented, the hybrid assessment model was more "knows how" than "shows how."

allows learners and teachers flexibility to make informed decisions about instructional changes [10]. The aim is to optimize student learning while understanding the limited time resources of teaching staff. Educators then need robust and reliable technology platforms that will not crash, as in **Case 10-2**, to allow remote assessment to develop to its potential. More stable platforms, debugged software, and much greater capacity (bandwidth and speed) are required to support this development.

Chapter 7 presented material relevant to computer-based tasting and artificial item generation, but these do not address the needs for new assessment methods that can assess domains other than knowledge and, to some extent, its application in brief written scenarios. If the concept of multiple methods, multiple judges, and multiple occasions is embraced, new assessment methods are required to complete a more holistic assessment of performance that demonstrates fitness to practice [11]. This includes interpreting larger blocks of text in a wide range of documents and safe observation of clinical practice. Assessment is likely to become more often adaptive, sequential, cumulative and accessible anywhere on mobile devices [12–14]. Technology will be at the center of these new methods because of the potential to facilitate measurement of a broad range of performance criteria as well as provide continuous on-demand testing and instantaneous feedback.

Another important lesson from this pandemic is that security measures need greater investment because the reported increase in internet fraud and crime could be redirected to assessment. Can hacking examination papers the night before high-stakes examinations be prevented? How confident are we that assessment item banks are protected from those who may want to acquire and sell mock examinations? Can we guarantee that confidentiality is protected and privacy is ensured for patients, candidates, and assessors? How can we strengthen proctoring and invigilating measures for online assessments, or should we cease proctoring, expand and release larger item banks, and adopt more widely open-book assessment methods? There may be an opportunity to develop more authentic assessment that better reflects how professionals maintain currency. Many of these changes were already inevitable, but the pandemic-influenced "leap" has accelerated development. On the other hand, could we go too far in the direction of technological adaptation, possibly predisposing medical education to a different kind of global disruption such as "failure" or corruption of the internet (satellite failure, prolonged solar storms) and the very technology that we see as a solution? In the recent 2020 report by the Joint Information Systems Committee on the future of assessment, educators are asked to embrace technology to transform assessment in five ways: Make it (1) more authentic by preparing the learner for using knowledge in practice or at work; (2) accessible, including to those with both short- and long-term disabilities or mental health issues; (3) appropriately automated, thereby easing teachers' marking and feedback workload and providing quicker, more detailed and more actionable feedback for students; (4) continuous, which is rich in practice opportunities and reflecting the fact that students today need to be capable of adapting to lifelong learning and the changing world of work; and (5) highly secure, discouraging cheating, and ensuring that the right student is taking the right assessment and that the work they are submitting is their own [15].

▌ CONCLUSION

The COVID-19 pandemic has posed substantial challenges to medical education because of the close integration of health and education services and the impact on broader societal functions of public health measures, such as enhanced hygiene, social distancing, and travel restrictions. The impact on clinical learning and assessment has been profound, yet medical educators have found ways to delay some assessments, accelerate other assessments for candidates near graduation, and vary or adapt the assessment methods used. The impact on accreditation in most cases has been a deferral for a year of accreditation activities and decisions. How long this disruption will last is difficult to predict, and some aspects of the disruption may persist as the 'new normal'. We may also need to prepare flexible approaches that may make the response to future major disruptions easier. Many of the adjustments made to assessment and its quality assurance require research to both build a stronger theoretical base and demonstrate effectiveness. New assessment methods may emerge. This disruption should be viewed as an opportunity to reflect on how assessment practices can be improved as well as made more sustainable.

▌ REFERENCES

1. Boursicot K, Kemp S, How Ong T, et al. Conducting a high-stakes OSCE in a COVID-19 environment. *MedEdPublish*. 2020. https://doi.org/10.15694/mep.2020.000054.1.
2. Wilkinson TJ, Smith JD, Margolis SA, Sen Gupta T, Prideaux DJ. Structured assessment using multiple patient scenarios by videoconference in rural settings. *Medical Education*. 2008;42(5):480–487.
3. Sen Gupta TK, Campbell D, Chater AB, et al. Fellowship of the Australian College of Rural & Remote Medicine (FACRRM) Assessment: A Review of the First 12 Years. *MedEdPublish*. 2020. https://doi.org/10.15694/mep.2020.000100.1
4. Bogossian F, Cant R, Cooper S, et al. Locating "gold standard" evidence for simulation as a substitute for clinical practice in pre-licensure health professional education: A systematic review. *Journal of Clinical Nursing*. 2019;28:3759–3775.
5. de Jong LH, Bok HG, Kremer WD, van der Vleuten CP. Programmatic assessment: Can we provide evidence for saturation of information? *Medical Teacher*. 2019;41(6):678–682.
6. Van Der Vleuten CPM, Schuwirth LWT. Assessing professional competence: From methods to programmes. *Medical Education*. 2005;39:309–317. https://doi.org/10.1111/j.1365-2929.2005.02094.x
7. Kichloo A, Albosta M, Dettloff K, et al. Telemedicine, the current COVID-19 pandemic and the future: A narrative review and perspectives moving forward in the USA. *Fam Med Community Health*. 2020 Aug;8(3):e000530. doi:10.1136/fmch-2020-000530. PMID: 32816942; PMCID: PMC7437610.
8. Black A. Gen Y: Who they are and how they learn. *Educational Horizons*. 2010; 88(2):92–101.
9. Reeves TC, Oh E. Generational Differences. *Handbook of Research on Educational Communications and Technology*. 2007;295–303.
10. Russell M. Technology-Aided Formative Assessment of Learning. In: Andrade HL, Cizek GJ, eds. *Handbook of Formative Assessment*. New York, NY: Routledge; 2010:125–138.

11. Batalden P, Leach D, Swing S, Dreyfus H, Dreyfus S. General competencies and accreditation in graduate medical education. *Health Aff* (Millwood). 2002Sep–Oct;21(5):103–111. doi:10.1377/hlthaff.21.5.103. PMID: 12224871

12. Homer MS, Fuller R, Pell G. The benefits of sequential testing: Improved diagnostic accuracy and better outcomes for failing students. *Medical Teacher*. 2018;40(3):275–284. https://doi.org/10.1080/0142159X.2017.1404561

13. Collares CF, Cecilio-Fernandes D. When I say … computerised adaptive testing. *Medical Education*. 2019;53(2):115–116. https://doi.org/10.1111/medu.13648

14. Triantafillou E, Georgiadou E, Economides A. The design and evaluation of a computerised adaptive test on mobile devices. *Computers & Evaluation*. 2008;50(4): 1319–1330. https://doi.org/10.1016/j.compedu.2006.12.005

15. Joint Information Systems Committee. (2020) The future of assessment: Five principles, five targets for 2025. https://www.jisc.ac.uk/reports/the-future-of-assessment

Glossary

Accreditation: A self-regulatory process by which governmental, nongovernmental, and voluntary associations or other statutory bodies grant formal recognition to educational programs or institutions that meet stated criteria of educational quality. Measurement against these standards includes reviews of written information, program self-studies, site visits to the educational program, and thoughtful consideration of the findings by a review committee. Whereas programs or institutions are accredited, individual physicians are licensed or certified.

Assessment: An evaluation or measurement of students' knowledge, skills, or attitude.

Assessment program: A mix of various assessment methods that are deliberately composed and appropriate for the aims, content, and structure of the curriculum.

Authenticity: A form of validity that refers to how similar an assessment is to the actual job that people are required to do or to the context in which they are required to do it.

Automated item generation: Item construction technology in which computer algorithms combine the elements of item models designed and developed by content specialists to produce a large number of test items in a short period of time.

Bias: The extent to which an assessment measures factors other than what it was designed to measure.

CanMEDS: Competency framework in health professions education.

Cognitive model: Structured framework containing the knowledge, skills, and content necessary to answer a test item; representation of the cognitive steps used by experts to approach a particular problem.

Computer-based testing (CBT): Tests administered with a computer, which implements processes to select and administer items. Students' performance is scored, and their ability in each item is categorized.

Criterion-referenced standard setting: Testing candidates against an absolute standard determined by examiner consensus, item performance data, or a combination of these sources.

Curriculum alignment: A process aimed at ensuring consistency between the intended learning outcomes, the planned and delivered curriculum, teaching and learning activities, and assessment content and processes for both classroom and workplace-based learning.

Edumetric perspective: From this perspective, tests are designed to detect student's learning and development. The tests yield scores that are meaningful without reference to the performance of others.

Electronic Portfolio (ePortfolio): That may include documents and aggregates and visualizes assessment data points, providing comprehensive overviews of the assessment data.

Equivalence of assessment: A broad term encompassing processes that lead to equivalent decisions being made as a result of assessments regardless of where or when they occurred.

External quality assurance: The systems that are designed and operated by an external agency (often mandated by law) to monitor the quality of education provided by higher education institutions.

Fairness: Impartial and just treatment or behavior without favoritism or discrimination.

False positive and **false negative results:** Sometimes candidates are able to answer a question correctly without having sufficient specific competence or, vice versa, the question leads them to provide an incorrect answer despite having sufficient specific competence. False positive and false negative results can occur at all levels; an individual item can generate a false positive and false negative answer, students can undeservedly pass fail a test, or students can even undeservedly pass or fail a whole year or a whole course.

Higher-order cognitive skills: Complex and iterative thinking processes that a candidate or student utilizes in producing the correct answer. This is a multistep process in which different pieces of information have to be considered and weighed against each other.

High-stakes examination: Examination that has major consequences for the test taker.

Internal quality assurance: The process of monitoring the teaching, learning, and assessment activities that a learner at a training provider will undertake.

Item bank: Pools of test items that contain information regarding their content and psychometric details.

Item format and **item stimulus:** Assessment items that can be characterized by their so-called stimulus and format. The *stimulus* refers to what the question asks, what is required of the candidate, and what we want the candidate to demonstrate. The *format* refers to how the candidate's response is captured.

Item model: General representation of the item to be generated that contain the elements that can be manipulated to create new items.

Learner, trainee, student: The person being observed through WBA.

Norm-referenced standard setting: Testing candidates against examination performance data of their peers (similar training and experience) on the same test.

Objective Structured Clinical Exams (OSCE): Used to assess clinical skills.

Program director, education leader: The leader of a curriculum.

Programmatic assessment: An assessment approach that aims to better align assessment with modern education—that is, competency-based education (see Chapter 6 for further information).

Progress test: An assessment method applied to longitudinally assess the cognitive domain.

Psychometric perspective: From this perspective, tests are designed to be able to discriminate between individual differences. The tests express results in terms of a norm.

Psychometrics: Quantitative measurement practices in psychology, education, and the social sciences; analyses aimed at determining the measurement quality of the assessment.

QA assessor: An individual appointed to investigate and report on the quality of assessment content, processes, and evaluations.

Quality assurance (QA): An inherent requirement and an ongoing, continuous process-oriented proactive evaluation approach to ensure the quality of assessment processes in medical education.

Quality improvement: The combined and unceasing efforts of everyone—health-care professionals, patients and their families, researchers, payers, planners. and educators—to make the changes that will lead to better patient outcomes (health), better system performance (care), and better professional development.

Reliability: The extent to which an assessment is reproducible or consistent.

Social accountability: For medical schools, this has been defined as the obligation to direct their education, research, and service activities toward addressing the priority health concerns of the community, region, or nation that they have a mandate to serve. The priority health concerns are to be identified jointly by governments, health-care organizations, health professionals, and the public.

Standard setting: The process that sets the passing score for an examination.

Supervisor, teacher, assessor, observer, rater: The person observing the performance of a learner through direct observation of the learner or their work.

Test form assembly (ATA): The process by which items in a particular assessment are arranged and presented to the test taker.

Test taker impairment: Permanent (e.g., dyslexia) or temporary (e.g., broken arm) factors that interfere with a person's ability to undertake or perform in a test other than the test taker's actual ability.

Test wiseness: The ability to respond advantageously to an assessment that is related to familiarity or ability with the test format rather than ability in the subject matter being tested.

Validity: The extent to which an assessment measures what it was designed to measure.

Very short answer question (VSAQ): Novel type of item consisting of a vignette followed by a question that requires candidates to generate short free-text responses.

Workplace-based assessment (WBA): The assessment of performance in practice, in-training assessment, and performance-based assessment.

Index

Page numbers followed by "t" denote tables; those followed by "f" denote figures; and those followed by "b" denote boxes.

265

www.ingramcontent.com/pod-product-compliance
Lightning Source LLC
Chambersburg PA
CBHW061340210326
41598CB00035B/5837